PATHFINDER
THE LIFE OF HARRIETTE CHICK

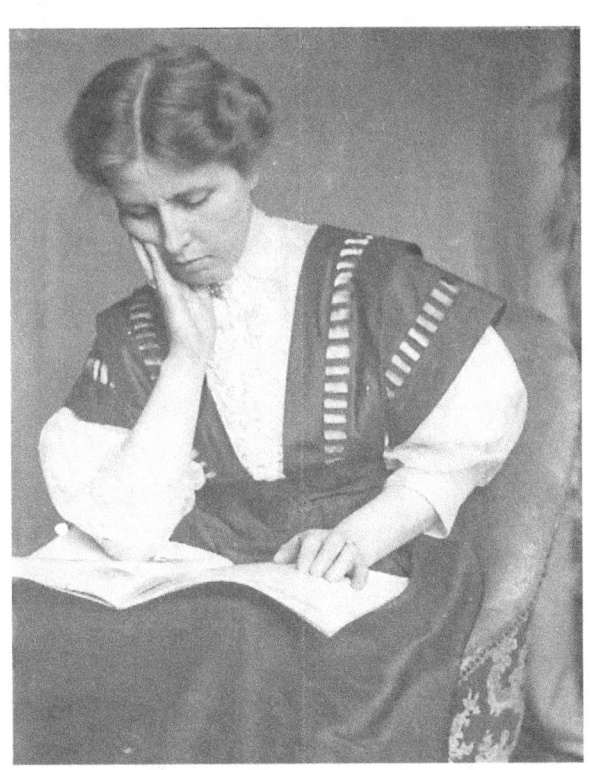

PATHFINDER

THE LIFE OF HARRIETTE CHICK

HOW THE STUDY OF VITAMINS BLAZED
A TRAIL FOR WOMEN IN SCIENCE

STEPHEN M. SAGAR, M.D.

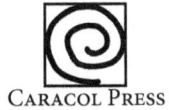

CARACOL PRESS

For permission requests, contact the author at sms@caracolpress.com

Published by Caracol Press
San Francisco, CA

Design by Kiran Spees

Cover photograph courtesy of National Portrait Gallery London.
Title page photograph courtesy of The Branscombe Project.

Library of Congress Control Number 2025904813
ISBN 979-8-9927895-0-8
e-book ISBN 979-8-9927895-1-5

For Susan and all the other
brave women who led the way.

The biographer of a scientist can expect to have the dubious pleasure of discovering that the obvious path which the subject would be expected to take was not the path that he took at all. And more importantly, the expected philosophical and social influences on his work are annoyingly complex and uncertain.

—Thomas L. Haskins (1979) In defense of biography: the use of biography in the history of science. *History of Science* 17: 1-16.

CONTENTS

PREFACE

Although few physicians have heard of Harriette Chick, she had a major role in medical science during the first half of the twentieth century. I knew nothing about her until I began doing research for my book *Vitamin C: A 500-Year Scientific Biography from Scurvy to Pseudoscience*. During World War I she performed some of the early laboratory studies of scurvy, the disease caused by vitamin C deficiency. Her meticulous experiments firmly established that scurvy was a nutritional disease at a time when many believed it to be a form of ptomaine poisoning from spoiled food.

As I read more, I came to realize that not only was the story of her scientific accomplishments important in the history of nutrition research, but she was also the first British woman in modern times to forge a career as a professional scientist, earning a salary and working as an equal alongside men in a major research institution. What was special about her and her circumstances that permitted her unique success?

At the turn of the twentieth century, British women were all but excluded from professional life and none were working as professional scientists. Some wealthy ladies conducted scientific research at their own, or their husbands', expense; others persisted despite limited resources. But even those who made significant discoveries were shut out of professional societies and had to enlist male colleagues to publish their work in scientific journals. Those who had the means and good fortune to attend secondary school and university could go on to earn an advanced degree in science, but were then relegated to teach school, serve as laboratory assistants, or marry and give up their careers altogether. By breaking out of this mold, Harriette Chick paved the way for the many talented women who followed.

My claim that she was the first is, of course, subject to challenge. In searching sources—published papers, histories of science, biographies of scientists, Wikipedia—I may have missed a woman who preceded her. Perhaps I did not look hard enough or in the right places. And there were a handful of women in Europe and the United States who were earning a salary as scientists. But whether Harriette Chick was first or fifth in Great Britain, she was an extremely unusual woman for her time and place.

The arc of her scientific career is notable in itself. She began her career as a bacteriologist and did some innovative experiments in the basic biochemistry of disinfectants. She could have gone on to a productive career in basic biochemistry but World War I intervened and she switched to nutrition research to support the war effort. There she made her most important discoveries, primarily in understanding vitamin deficiency diseases. Besides her work on scurvy, her studies of tropical beriberi saved countless British soldiers from the disease after she advised the army to add yeast extract to their rations.

However, it was her work on rickets in Vienna after World War I that cemented her status as a leader in medical science. Rickets, caused by vitamin D deficiency, was then a common disease in polluted, dark industrial cities, stunting the growth of children and deforming bones. Harriette Chick's work led to a generation of children being given cod liver oil and, later, the enrichment of milk with vitamin D. As a result, rickets virtually disappeared from the developed world, a major contribution to medical science and to public health.

But her very success led to her name being forgotten. She is not mentioned in medical school lectures, which describe rickets as a disease of merely historical importance. If you search Wikipedia for *female scientists in the 20th century*, her name does not appear. What is also forgotten, along with her scientific contributions, is her role as a pioneer for women in science. Women continue to face barriers in pursuing careers in science, where leadership positions are still dominated by men. But thanks to Harriette Chick and her fellow pioneers, the door was opened. This book is a tribute to her courage and accomplishments.

CHAPTER 1
THE BOSS'S FOLLY

In 1904, Harriette Chick found herself at a crossroads. Then 29 years old, she had aspired to be a scientist since high school and had just taken a big step, receiving her D.Sc. degree in bacteriology from the University of London. But she did not know how she would exploit this prestigious credential to forge a career. She had no role models. Women of her era did not concern themselves with their careers, since they were generally barred from professional jobs. Proper British ladies did not earn money; they could only marry into it.

But Harriette had no interest in becoming a housewife. For the previous two years, aside from a period in Munich finishing up a research project, she had lived with her family in Ealing, a neighborhood of west London, and worked as an assistant to Dr. A.C. Houston, a bacteriologist for the Royal Commission on Sewage Disposal, monitoring bacterial contamination of London water. The work was important to the public health, but uninteresting. Harriette was little more than a laboratory technician. Overqualified for the job, she aspired to put her degree to better use. The Chick family had a heritage of ambitious women and Harriette aspired to do more than routine work.

She had obtained her undergraduate degree from University College London (UCL) where she excelled, the only student in her class to earn honors in botany. Each English university nominated one outstanding graduate each year for an 1851 Exhibition Scientific Research Scholarship to support graduate research.* UCL nominated Harriette Chick in 1899. With the scholarship, she went to work with Prof. Rupert Boyce, an expert in public health at the recently opened Thompson-Yates Laboratories of University College Liverpool.† This proved to be a momentous decision, but only indirectly due to Prof. Boyce.

The laboratories occupied a new, three-story building. The ground floor and basement housed the Pathology Department led by Dr. Boyce. The Physiology Department, headed by the eminent neurophysiologist Charles Sherrington, occupied the upper two floors. As was to be key to her future, Harriette became friendly with her upstairs neighbor, occasionally helping out in his laboratory.

In Boyce's laboratory, Harriette continued her study of bacteriology. She had a productive year, publishing a paper describing the metabolism of a species of algae that she had cultured from a polluted pond. The 1851 Exhibition Commission renewed her scholarship for a second year, allowing her to move to Vienna to work with another expert in public health, Max von Gruber, with whom she studied the bacteriology of sewage treatment. After the year in Vienna, she returned to London, moved back in with her parents and two sisters. and took the job with Dr. Houston. She submitted her work in Liverpool as her doctoral thesis.

Once she had her doctorate, Sherrington urged her to apply for the Jenner Memorial Research Studentship at the Lister Institute of Preventive Medicine in London. Sherrington, a keen judge of talent, strongly recommended her to his friend Charles Martin, the Director of the Lister Institute: "I believe her an accomplished bacteriologist...Personally I know her quite well, and should describe her as clever, hardworking, enthusiastic, and moreover a person of culture."[1]

Founded in 1891, the Lister Institute under Martin's leadership was on its way to becoming the pre-eminent medical research facility in Great Britain.

---

* The 1851 Exhibition, the first world's fair, generated over £200,000 in profit. The funds were used to buy land in the Kensington district of London for a number of institutions (Imperial College, the Victoria and Albert Museum, the Royal Albert Hall and the Natural History Museum, among others) and to endow scholarships and fellowships in scientific research. These grants are still being awarded.

† Now the University of Liverpool.

The Jenner Research Studentship had been endowed by Edward Guinness, Lord Iveagh, the owner of the Guinness brewery and the major benefactor of the Lister Institute. It was a prestigious award intended to support young scientists on their way to membership on the faculty of the Institute. The Studentship offered Harriette an opportunity to do original research mentored by some of the best scientists in Great Britain and could be a start on the path to the career she desired. However, it was a reach. The previous recipients had all been men and the professional staff of the Institute were all men as well.

The Institute's major focus was infectious diseases. With her background in bacteriology and public health, stellar academic record, and letter of recommendation from Charles Sherrington, Harriette was the perfect candidate—except for her gender. Two members of the staff strenuously objected to her appointment, urging Dr. Martin not to "commit the folly" of appointing a woman to the position.[2] Since they assumed that she would be unable to have her own career, giving her the Studentship would waste a valuable resource.

But Martin valued the advice of Charles Sherrington, one of Great Britain's most distinguished scientists, more than the prejudices of some of his colleagues. He not only committed the folly of awarding Harriette the Jenner Memorial Research Studentship, he took her on in his laboratory. With Sherrington's encouragement and help, she had found more interesting work than monitoring London's water. And she had found a mentor in Dr. Martin, *the Boss* as she and her colleagues called him, who remained a collaborator, champion, and close friend throughout her career.

She and Martin began their collaboration by carrying out groundbreaking experiments on the biochemistry of disinfectants, establishing Harriette's credentials as an original investigator. After the chilly welcome, Harriette rapidly proved her mettle and was "soon accepted on terms of equality and friendship by the apprehensive males."[3] When the Studentship ended after two years, she advanced to full membership on the scientific staff.

This was a landmark achievement. Harriette Chick became England's first female professional scientist since the eighteenth century to obtain a permanent, salaried position.* Few women in the world had achieved that status.

---

* Caroline Herschel (1750-1848), sister of the famous astronomer William Herschel, in 1787 was granted an annual salary of £50 by King George III to work as William's assistant.

Several British women had preceded her in obtaining graduate and postgraduate training in science, but for the most part they either married and gave up any chance of a career or they became secondary schoolteachers. A few had university teaching positions. Harriette Chick was first to launch a career as an independent investigator, going on to make many contributions to medical science with substantial impacts on public health. Her success paved the way for the women who followed.

The story of how Harriette Chick established herself in a profession that was dominated by men and rife with sexism began three generations earlier with Harriette's great-grandmother, Abigail Chick. Harriette was not the first trailblazer among the Chick women

Notes

1   Letter dated 13 March 1905, archives of the Wellcome Library, London.

2   Chick, Harriette; Hume, Margaret; and Macfarlane, Marjorie (1971) *War on Disease. A History of the Lister Institute* (London: Andre Deutsch), p. 88.

3   Chick H et al. (1971) *War on Disease,* p. 88.

CHAPTER 2
HONITON LACE

Harriette's niece, Margaret Tomlinson, in 1985 published the Chick family history in *Three Generations in the Honiton Lace Trade*.[1] Her account begins in the eighteenth century, when her ancestors were tenant farmers in Somerset and Devon, a quiet agricultural region in the southwest of England. Farms spread over a countryside dotted with small towns. The inhabitants enjoyed a warmer climate than the rest of England and were spared the polluted air of the industrial north.

The land was almost all owned by absentee landlords, either landed gentry living off the rents or by the Dean and Chapter, the governing body and business arm of the local diocese of the Church of England. Yeoman farmers, like the Chicks, who had accumulated enough capital to afford the leases could make a good living and enjoy a middle-class lifestyle. Below them on the economic ladder was a large class of impoverished farm workers paid barely enough to survive. Somerset and Devon were among the poorest regions of England.

Although this hardly appears to have been fertile ground to nurture entrepreneurs, Harriette's great-grandmother Abigail became just that. Born in 1778, she was the seventh and youngest child of William Tutcher and Sara Vincent of Buckland St. Mary in Somerset. Sara was illiterate, unable to sign her own name in the marriage registry; but Abigail likely attended grammar school and could read, write, and do arithmetic.

We do not know how she met her husband, Samuel Chick, the son of tenant farmers in Axminster, about twenty-five miles from Buckland St. Mary. When Samuel and Abigail married in 1804, they moved to Branscombe, a sleepy seaside village of about 600 inhabitants where Samuel leased farmland. Houses lined a road running parallel to the coast, and farms spread to either side over rolling hills. A side road ran down to lime kilns and the beach. The village now attracts vacationers but has not markedly changed in appearance or grown in population since Samuel and Abigail arrived.

Samuel first leased land on the western edge of the village from a local landowner, John Stuckey, the wealthiest man in Branscombe. Samuel later expanded his holdings, leasing his largest tracts from the Dean and Chapter. His leasehold eventually totaled several hundred acres. He was a prosperous farmer and an important member of the community.

However, according to her grandson Elijah, Abigail's constitution was "far too restless to allow her to sit down quietly in the humdrum life of a farm."[2] A silhouette from about 1835 shows a woman to be reckoned with: straight-backed in a full skirt, peering down her nose at a book held in her hand, perhaps her ledger. She not only raised a family but also founded a lace business that supported the Chicks for the next century.

Devon had become the center of lace making in England, producing a style called *Honiton lace*, named after a village in East Devon. In the sixteenth century, Flemish refugees brought the technique of *pillow lace* or *bobbin lace* across the Channel. Fashionable English consumers generally preferred French and Belgian lace; but the Napoleonic Wars disrupted the Continental lace industry, allowing Devon to become a major producer.

Lace was made "by the poor, for the rich."[3] It was the model cottage industry. Young women, usually in their teens, apprenticed to lace-making schools. After mastering the techniques, they worked in their own homes. They required little equipment: a straw-stuffed canvas pillow; some pins to affix a pattern and the lace fragment to the pillow; and bobbins, wooden dowels used to manipulate the threads to form lace.

Each worker made fragments called *sprigs*. The lace dealer provided patterns and thread to the workers and then collected the sprigs and leftover thread, which was weighed to be sure the workers were not hoarding it for their own use. The dealer assembled the sprigs into finished garments, which they sold in their own shop or to other retailers. With diligent work, a lace maker could earn the equivalent of a shilling per day, close to the wage of a farm laborer. However, many dealers paid them in trade goods rather than currency, a source of resentment among the workers.

Abigail recognized her opportunity to enter this business, which required little capital but a lot of energy. She enlisted a panel of lace workers and established herself as likely the only female lace dealer in Devon. Even more remarkable for a woman of her time, she traveled on her own throughout Great Britain and occasionally to the Continent to buy and sell lace. Although hers was not the largest lace business in Devon, by the 1830s it had grown into a substantial enterprise.

In addition to being hardworking, the Chicks were religious. By 1824, Samuel and Abigail had become Wesleyan Methodists. Although the Church of England remained dominant, Methodism had grown in importance in Devon. John Wesley had spent time there, preaching his interpretation of the scriptures. After his death in 1791, his followers split from the Church of England. Methodism then achieved its greatest growth among miners and factory workers in the north of England, but it also made inroads in the southwest among the middle class. The warm climate and scenic, rural landscape made Devon a favorite destination for itinerant Methodist preachers, giving them a break from the dark, polluted skies and urban slums of the north.

Methodism appealed to yeoman farmers by being more egalitarian than the Church of England, giving lay men and even lay women a role in managing the churches and conducting services. Most Anglicans thought that only the wealthy could enter Heaven, since, in their minds, poverty was invariably associated with moral depravity. In contrast, any Methodist, even the poorest laborer, could find salvation by having faith in Christ and leading a righteous life. At the same time, Methodism justified paying workers as little as possible to shield them from the temptations of materialism.

Methodist *societies*, the equivalent of congregations, provided social life in rural towns and for urban laborers too poor to attend the theater or host dinner parties. Samuel was likely a founder of the Branscombe society in 1815. In 1831, he and twenty-three other men built the first Methodist chapel in Branscombe and later replaced it with a larger structure on a different site.*

After building her business, Abigail retired in 1848 at age 70, and she and Samuel moved to Sidmouth. Samuel died in 1851, leaving Abigail an estate of over £4,000 (equivalent to about £700,000 today). Five years later, Abigail married Joseph Gray, a widower from the nearby village of Sidbury and also a Wesleyan Methodist. She died in 1858 and was buried next to Samuel in Sidmouth. Her remarkable life established a precedent for Chick women and the stories of her success were passed down to her descendants.

Samuel and Abigail had four children, two daughters and two sons. The elder son, Samuel, born in 1811, was never robust and had a deformed leg that made it impossible for him to operate a farm. He was good with his hands, however, and went to Weymouth to learn watchmaking. A portrait shows him in profile, wearing a top hat and long sideburns, riding along the Weymouth waterfront in a dog-propelled wheelchair he designed and probably built himself. He married his first cousin, Harriet Staple, in 1845. They opened a lace shop in Weymouth and took over Abigail's business when she retired. Samuel's poor health made it likely that Harriet followed Abigail's example and ran the business. In 1849, Samuel and Harriet hired a woman to operate the shop in Weymouth and moved to Sidmouth, where they could be closer to their workers.

Their older daughter, Harriet Ann, married John Tucker. The Tuckers had their own lace business, which was even more successful than the Chicks'. John ran their business and by 1851 he was the largest employer in the region. The Tuckers and Chicks became business rivals for a time; but when John Tucker died in 1877, his business closed while the Chicks' continued. This allowed the families to resume a close relationship.

The 1850s marked the peak in demand for Honiton lace, when there were thousands of women in East Devon employed in the craft. However, with relative peace on the Continent and changes in fashion, the demand for Honiton

---

* That structure still exists but has been converted to residences.

lace declined and the lace business may have become insufficient to support the Chick family. To fill the gap, Samuel and Harriet took on other businesses, including an inn in Sidmouth. Following his parents' tradition, Samuel was active in the local Wesleyan Methodist community.

The couple had five children, three boys and two girls. The older boy, born in 1841, was the third Samuel in the line and would become Harriette's father. He and his brother attended a Wesleyan boarding school in Taunton. Samuel hated it, especially geometry; but he stuck it out and graduated. Imbued with the strong religious faith of his family, Samuel aspired to be a minister. However, his mother persuaded him to take over the family lace business instead. To prepare for a career selling fabrics, he briefly apprenticed to drapers in Cheltenham. Despite giving up his desire to enter the clergy, he remained deeply religious throughout his life.

Samuel met Emma Hooley in 1862 when he was twenty-one, she eighteen. Emma was the daughter of a Methodist corn merchant and grocer in Macclesfield in the north of England. She and her sister took the train to Devon to visit an uncle, who had recently moved to Newton Poppleford, seven miles from Sidmouth, to set up a wool mill. Getting word of the visit through their Methodist connections, the Chick boys were only too happy to ride out to the nearby station to welcome the young women and help with their luggage.

Samuel immediately began wooing Emma. For unknown reasons, Emma's parents did not welcome him as a suitor, whereas the Chicks were enthusiastic about the match from the start. Emma had not a hair out of place, according to her future mother-in-law. A photograph of her as a young woman verifies that description. She looked almost exactly like Harriette at a similar age. Although it took a few years, the Hooleys eventually warmed up to Samuel and came to appreciate him as a serious young man with excellent business sense.

In 1863, Samuel moved to London to expand the family's lace business. He set up a shop and warehouse at 5 Newman Street in the Fitzrovia district, just around the corner from the fashionable Oxford Street shops and convenient for well-off shoppers.* The terraced house had showrooms on the first floor and living quarters above. Samuel's sister Harriet sent him lace designs, and his mother and his brother Edward helped manage the manufacturing in Devon. His father kept the books and invoiced the customers. In addition to selling to the London market, Samuel traveled throughout England to market his wares. He was always eager to go to the north, where he could see Emma. Although he did not feel welcome at the Hooleys, he would meet her at one of her friend's house.

Samuel became a Baptist and a deacon of the Regents Park Baptist Chapel. As a young man he was a teetotaler. Politically he was a Liberal, secretary of the Marylebone Liberal Association and a member of the Passive Resistance League, an ill-fated effort to protest taxes that supported the Church of England. His business, at first hand-to-mouth, eventually did well enough that, having overcome the Hooleys' reservations, he and Emma married in 1867.

Emma joined Samuel at 5 Newman Street to begin a long and happy marriage. They had complementary personalities. "Emma was prudent, practical and rather solemn, while Samuel was overflowing with energy, always impatient to be up and doing."[4] Emma restrained some of his impetuous instincts and calmed him down when he became irritated with his business partners, his sister Harriet or his brother Edward. Samuel expanded his territory to buying and selling lace from the Continent. Emma sometimes accompanied him on trips abroad, providing advice on the latest styles.

With changes in fashion, Samuel's income from selling lace declined; but he had accumulated enough capital to begin buying commercial properties in the area around his shop on Newman Street. He focused his investments on the area he knew well and proved adept at the real estate business. He soon was gaining most of his income from rents.

The family was comfortably middle-class, although in the English class system they were "in trade" and therefore considered inferior to titled aristocrats, the landed gentry and the professional class. Being Nonconformists, that is, not members of the Church of England, further distanced them from

---

* The building no longer exists, having been replaced by a more modern mixed-use structure.

London society. Samuel's social life centered on his work, his church, and the Liberal Association. Emma devoted her energy to her house, her husband, and her growing family.

Notes

1   Tomlinson, Margaret (1985) *Three Generations in the Honiton Lace Trade.* Sidmouth, Devon: Sovereign Printing Group.

This book recounts the Chick family history through 1925 and is the source of that information for this and much of the following chapter. Margaret Tomlinson was the daughter of Harriette's oldest sister Edith. For her book, she recorded the reminiscences of her mother and aunts. Moreover, she was intimately familiar with the towns in Devon from whence the Chicks hailed; and she combed their parish and municipal records.

Like Harriette and other Chick women, Margaret forged a successful career. Born in 1905, she studied architecture at Cambridge. She married and had two children; but the marriage broke up in 1941, leaving her a single mother needing work. She moved to Devon to be near her family and found a job as a photographer with the National Buildings Record, a program to preserve images of historic buildings threatened by the war. Some of her photographs are striking (https://historicengland.org.uk/ research/inclusive-heritage/womens-history/women-photographers-in-historic-en- gland-archive/margaret-tomlinson/). They are beautifully composed, the prints technically excellent. After the war she worked in city planning and published her family history in 1985. She died in 1997 at age 92.

2   Tomlinson M (1985) *Three Generations*, p. 18.

3   https://laceincontext.com/

4   Tomlinson M (1985) *Three Generations*, p. 64.

CHAPTER 3
GROWING UP

In 1868 Emma gave birth to twins, a boy, the fourth Samuel Chick, and a girl, Alice, who died at birth. Samuel and Emma went on to have ten more children, nine of whom survived to adulthood.

None of their three sons made their mark in the world. The eldest, Samuel IV, was the biggest disappointment. He was reckless with money, women, and drink. He had only a brief marriage, failed in business, and never became financially independent. Edward, born in 1871, died of appendicitis at age twenty-six. We know little of James except that he was born in 1880, survived service in World War I, never married, and died in 1933.

Although the British upper classes considered it inappropriate for a lady to earn money, Samuel and Emma did not suffer from this bias. A heritage of productive women contributing to the family's income made the Chicks unusual for their time in assuming that their daughters could have careers other than as housewives. Especially since their sons showed little promise, they invested in their daughters' education. Of the seven daughters, five graduated from university. Besides Harriette, the two youngest were the most accomplished: Frances, whose married surname was Wood, became a statistician of note. The Royal Statistical Society awards the Wood Medal every three years in her honor.* Dorothy became a surgeon. Both died in their thirties of acute infections.

---

* The web page of the Society states: The Wood Medal was established in memory of the

Harriette, born in 1875, was the fifth child and third daughter to survive infancy. She spent her childhood in London during the school year and her summers in Devon. The time in London was like being in jail, subject to her father's rigorous discipline. Samuel was a strict father and a strict Baptist. Although he had not realized his ambition of becoming a minister, he conducted family prayers morning and evening. On Sundays, the children attended two church services plus Sunday school. He banned worldly entertainments including theater and dancing. Emma deferred to her husband in matters of the children's discipline.

Furthermore, Samuel and Emma were not demonstrably affectionate parents. As Margaret Tomlinson wrote, "Samuel and Emma, so devoted to one another, appeared as remote and unapproachable figures to their growing children."[1] Emma loved infants and for over a decade could dote on one after another; but she grew distant as they grew older.

The summers in Devon gave the children a welcome release from their father's yoke. Initially they stayed with their grandmother Harriet in the town of Sidmouth, crowded into her house with her unmarried brother Edward and a varying number of young cousins. Their grandmother, like their mother, was not openly affectionate; but she allowed the children complete freedom as long as they showed up promptly for meals. They enjoyed exploring the fields and swimming at the beach with their friends and cousins. They had to endure only a single Methodist service on Sundays and even got to go to the circus. Their uncle Edward enjoyed their company. He was a good musician and piqued their interest in science by showing them the stars through his telescope and entertaining them with chemistry experiments.

After grandmother Harriet died in 1892, the children spent their summers in Branscombe. Two girls, generally the youngest, stayed with their cousins, the five Miss Tuckers. The older children stayed in a nearby rented cottage with the older girls looking after their younger siblings. That the cottage, free from adult oversight, was the preferred accommodation was a source of sibling resentment.

In 1901, Samuel rented Hazelwood, a seven-bedroom house on the side

---

statistician Frances Wood OBE (1883–1919). It is awarded every three years to a fellow of the Society for excellent contributions to economic or social statistics.

of a hill overlooking Branscombe. It became the summer residence for the family. Like all houses in Branscombe at the time, it lacked running water and indoor plumbing; but it had panoramic views and beautiful grounds, which climbed the hillside behind the house and stables. All the Chicks grew to love that house. After Samuel died in 1925, his children continued to rent it. When the owner died five years later, the Chick daughters bought the property from the estate and added to its grounds over the years. It remained with the family until the 1970s when Harriette donated it to the National Trust.*

The Gower Street School

In gaining an education, Harriette had two great advantages: her parents could afford to send her to private schools and they wanted their daughters to have a solid education. But she had two disadvantages: girls had limited educational opportunities and her family was Nonconformist. She had the good luck to have access to schools that pioneered in serving both groups.

Her grammar school, the Gower Street School for Girls, was within walking distance of the house on Newman Street. It was the successor to the Bedford College School, founded in 1849 to prepare girls for college. But the nondenominational school closed in 1868 when its trustees feared that the headmaster was trying to make it Anglican. One of its teachers, Lucy Harrison, a Quaker, then opened the Gower Street School, a *dame school*, a private grammar school supported by tuition. The four oldest Chick daughters attended. They learned, according to Harriette, "some arithmetic, languages 'fairly well,' a lot of poetry by heart, and how to speak."[2]

Harriette progressed through primary school and, at the age of twelve, graduated to the Notting Hill High School in the Bayswater area of London. She could no longer walk to school and had to take the Underground, a daunting prospect at first. The carriages were still drawn by steam locomotives; and the fumes in the tunnels were noxious, "a form of mild torture which no person would undergo if he could conveniently help it," according to *The Times*.[3] Nevertheless, the move set her on her way to a career. The Notting

---

* After being renovated, it is now leased out but still known by some of the locals as "Dame Harriette Chick's place." However, when I knocked on the door, the teenage girl who answered knew nothing about a previous resident named Harriette Chick.

Hill High School was one of the first in Great Britain to teach mathematics and science to girls. Its founding in 1873 encapsulates the story of secondary education for girls in Victorian England.

The Notting Hill High School

Prior to the second half of the nineteenth century, British girls had limited educational opportunities after grammar school. Wealthy families engaged tutors for their daughters; but middle-class girls had few choices except to attend one of the many private schools that prepared them to be governesses, the only occupation aside from housewife or prostitution generally available to them. In the 1851 census, there were 24,770 governesses in England. Their education, inconsistent in quality, focused on music, French, and needlework. Founded in 1841, the Governesses' Benevolent Association offered more rigorous training than that available in the private schools.

F. D. Maurice, a professor at King's College, began conducting evening classes for governesses to expose them to literature and the arts. He then founded Queen's College in 1848, a secondary school for girls aged eleven to eighteen. The curriculum included the same subjects taught to boys, attracting criticism for teaching mathematics to girls. It was commonly believed that their brains were not suited to rigorous thought. The Bedford College for Women, founded a year later to provide higher education to women, faced the problem that there were too few well-prepared women students to permit a true university level of instruction. The Bedford College School, the precursor of the Gower Street School, like Queen's College, tried to address that issue.

The Endowed Schools Commission was formed in 1864 to improve English secondary education for both boys and girls. *Endowed schools* were private secondary schools supported by wealthy benefactors. Some charged modest tuition and others were free. Most were day schools. They attracted students from middle-class families and their curriculum was more practical than that of what the British term public schools—Eton, Harrow, Westminster and the like—boarding schools that catered to the aristocracy and focused on the classics.

In 1867, the Commission issued a report that recommended that endowed schools provide the same education to girls as to boys. The report pointed out the inequality of resources: the endowment for boys' schools totaled £177,000 per year compared to £3,000 for girls. Accordingly, 36,874 boys were attending these secondary schools and only 113 girls.

To address this discrepancy, in 1871 a group of wealthy women formed the Women's Educational Union. One of the founders, Miss Emily Shirreff, wrote of the schools for governesses: "...girls are taught anyhow, and often not at all, acquiring scraps of flimsy information with a little bad French and worse music, at a cost heavy to the parents and utterly insufficient to give fair remuneration to the teachers. To attempt a remedy for this evil is the fixed purpose of the Union."[4] To develop a pipeline of qualified teachers, the Union drafted an education curriculum and opened the College for Training Women Teachers.

In 1872, led by Emily Shirreff and her sister, Maria Grey, members of the Union formed the Girls' Public Day School Company* to operate nondenominational secondary schools for girls. The curriculum was to mirror that of boys' schools and include mathematics, science, history, music, and modern languages. They raised barely enough money, much of which was donated by Miss Shirreff, to open two schools, one at Notting Hill north of Hyde Park and the other in Chelsea south of the Park. The Notting Hill High School prospered while the one in Chelsea floundered.

Harriet Morant Jones, the first headmistress of the Notting Hill High School, made it a success. Miss Jones grew up and taught school on the Isle of Guernsey. At first reluctant to move to London, she finally agreed to take on the post and, along with one other teacher, opened the Notting Hill High School on September 16, 1873. The building, a former boys' school, was dominated by one large hall, the classes separated only by curtains. The ten pioneering pupils ranged from five to fifteen years old. At most two had attended school before, others having been taught at home by governesses.

Although Miss Jones was an excellent administrator, she was not a scholar and received mixed reviews as a teacher. Within months she had recruited Marion Andrews, a graduate of Bedford College for Women, to lead the academic program. Ms. Andrews taught Latin, geometry, political economy and physics, winning the universal admiration of her students. She attracted members of the first generation of women graduates of the universities of London, Oxford, and Cambridge to bolster the teaching staff. The quality of teaching was excellent. By

* Now the Girl's Day School Trust, which operates 25 schools educating 20,000 girls.

the 1880s, the student body had grown to between fifty and sixty students, many from wealthy Nonconformist families in nearby Bloomsbury.

Two Strong-Willed Women

Harriette owed her good fortune in attending this innovative school to two determined women: her oldest sister Edith and Lady Stanley of Alderley.

When Edith finished grammar school at Gower Street at age sixteen, Samuel assumed that she would enter the family lace business. Edith had a different plan. She wanted to be a teacher and she let her father know that she was determined to follow her own path. Samuel was not used to opposition by women in his family. His wife Emma was no pushover, but she did not openly defy her husband. She was a peacemaker by nature. Presumably, she brokered a truce between Edith and Samuel.

Samuel, to his credit, acceded to Edith's desires and searched for a way to allow her to pursue her chosen career. His friends in the local Liberal Association referred him to Lady Henrietta Stanley, one of the founders of the Girls' Public Day School Company. Lady Stanley was a formidable woman. Her grandson, Bertrand Russell, was afraid of her. "She had a caustic tongue, and spared neither age nor sex."[5] He described her as "always downright, free from prudery and eighteenth century rather than Victorian in her conversation."[6] Her passions were science, about which she read widely, Italy, where she had grown up, and women's education. She had been instrumental in the 1869 founding of Girton College, the first women's college of Cambridge University, where her portrait still hangs.

Lady Stanley lived in a mansion near Buckingham Palace in the Mayfair district of London. Like a proper woman of her time, she spent her afternoons entertaining visitors in her drawing room and granted Samuel an audience. She immediately displayed her sharp tongue, telling Samuel "You people send your daughters to cheap schools and then expect us to accept them when it is too late to repair the damage."[7] By "you people" she meant those in trade and by "us" she meant those with inherited money and titles.

Samuel was not as easily intimidated as the young Bertrand Russell. He pointed out that the tuition at the Gower Street School was hardly cheap. He might also have added that the Gower Street School focused on academic subjects, whereas aristocratic young ladies spent much of their school day practicing social deportment and ballroom dancing. Lady Stanley softened and suggested he speak with Miss Jones at the Notting Hill High School.

Miss Jones had personal charisma as well as administrative skills. According to Harriette, Samuel and Emma immediately became "totally subjected" to her; and Miss Jones remained a lifelong friend of the Chick family.[8] Beginning with Edith, all seven Chick daughters attended Notting Hill High School and five graduated. Mary, the second oldest, left because of ill health and entered the family lace business instead of Edith. Margaret, the next in line after Harriette, left to become a teacher of elocution.

In 1887, Harriette easily passed her entrance exam for the Notting Hill High School. About this time, Samuel bought a large house in Ealing and moved his family to the more spacious quarters with a half-acre yard and views of downtown London. And the commute for his daughters to school was a ten-minute ride along a suburban route of the Underground, a much easier ride than the trip from the heart of London.

Harriette blossomed. She progressed up the academic track for students aspiring to go on to university. She enjoyed Latin, mathematics and science, especially biology. Her favorite teacher was Mary Adamson, a graduate of UCL, who taught science. Harriette graduated in 1893 at age eighteen. Later in life, she had fond memories of her secondary school years and remained in touch with Miss Jones. Most importantly, the Notting Hill High School gave her a love for science and hopes for a career.

University and Postgraduate Training

Following in the footsteps of her teacher, Ms. Andrews, Harriette enrolled in the Bedford College for Women in Marylebone in central London. Elizabeth Jesser Reid, a wealthy activist, founded the college in 1851 as the first institution of higher education in Great Britain exclusively for women. When Mrs. Reid died in 1866, she left an endowment for the Reid Trust to provide scholarships for students at Bedford College; Harriette Chick won one.

She entered college seeking to continue her studies of science and mathematics, her interests nurtured at Notting Hill High School. However, although strong in arts and literature, Bedford College was weak in mathematics and science. Harriette stayed only one year; in 1894, she relinquished the Reid Scholarship and transferred to UCL.

UCL was founded in 1826 as the University of London and admitted its first class of 641 students in 1828. While the venerable universities of Oxford and Cambridge only granted degrees to members of the Church of England, the University of London was militantly nonsectarian. It admitted Nonconformists, Jews and Catholics. It had no chapel, it banned religious instruction on its premises, and it did not allow clergy to hold faculty appointments. Anglicans called it "that godless institution on Gower Street."

The University of London committed two other sins that earned the disdain of the Oxbridge elite. Because it aimed to educate the middle class, the Whig press spurned it as "the Cockney college." Plus, it taught practical subjects, including medicine, science, engineering, studio art, and modern foreign languages. The universities at Oxford and Cambridge catered to the sons of the aristocracy, teaching them dead languages and equally moribund philosophy along with a little mathematics. No gentleman would deign to study anything that suggested he might someday have to earn a living.

Besides earning the opposition of the Church of England and Oxford and Cambridge Universities, the London medical establishment lined up against the upstart school. Their private, hospital-based medical schools did not welcome competition from a university. The Whig government refused to grant a Royal Charter. Without a charter, the University of London could not award degrees and had trouble attracting students.

By 1836 some of the founders of the University had gained influence in the government and a charter was finally granted. The name was changed to University College London and a separate charter was granted for a new entity which assumed the name of University of London. This new University of London was purely administrative, taking on responsibility for several affiliated colleges, including UCL and Bedford. The University of London conducted examinations and granted degrees, while the affiliated colleges did the teaching. This awkward system persisted until 1905, when UCL attained full responsibility for educating and examining its students while the University of London continued to grant the degrees.

In addition to being nondenominational, UCL introduced many other innovations in English education. From its inception, it emulated German universities and the University of Edinburgh in basing its teaching on lectures by specialists in a field rather than the Oxbridge system of tutors. In 1830 it opened a boys' school, "one of the earliest schools to attempt to dissociate education and flogging."[9] In the 1840s it built the world's first chemistry teaching laboratory where students could perform their own experiments.

Beginning in 1868, UCL admitted women. At first, the women's classes were segregated in their own building; but that proved too cumbersome and by 1878 all classes except medicine and life drawing were mixed. Like the men, women earned University of London degrees.

Harriette thrived at UCL. She continued to excel in mathematics and biology. She won the advanced-class prize in botany and the senior class Gold Medal. She received her B.S. degree in 1896 and progressed to postgraduate work in the sciences. With the germ theory at the cutting edge of medical science, she took courses in bacteriology and analytical chemistry from 1896 to 1899.

In 1899 she won the 1851 Exhibition Research Scholarship and chose to go to Liverpool to work with Prof. Rupert Boyce in the Thompson-Yates Laboratories. This was a promising opportunity for a burgeoning microbiologist. The newly constructed facilities of the Thompson-Yates Laboratories were among the most modern in the world. Boyce, a medical graduate of UCL and the most prominent British expert on public health and tropical medicine, had just assumed an endowed chair of pathology.

Harriette took up the study of wastewater. Why would a prim, upper middle-class young woman choose to study polluted water? Because Londoners were preoccupied by filth.[10] The streets were covered in mud and horse manure; the air stank of animal waste; stagnant water nurtured microorganisms and added to the bad odors. Throughout her career, Harriette took her scientific curiosity to where she found a pressing need. Microorganisms in the environment and their role in health were little understood. She saw it as an important problem with the potential to impact public health. In addition, she had the opportunity to learn from one of the most prominent scientists in Europe.

With Prof. Boyce, Chick investigated algae in polluted waters. Algae had attracted little scientific study. Microbiology had focused on bacteria and their role in diseases. Unlike bacteria, algae are plants, as they contain chlorophyll. Harriette focused on their nitrogen metabolism, as nitrogenous substances in urine and feces support the growth of microorganisms that render polluted water smelly and unhealthy. She wanted to better understand the biochemistry of these foul waters, in particular how microorganisms convert simple molecules into more complex substances that render the water unhealthy.

Harriette isolated a species of algae from pond water and christened it *Chlorella pyrenoidosa*. She measured its rate of growth and described its microscopic appearance when cultured under a variety of conditions. She showed that it could metabolize simple nitrogenous substances, such as ammonia, urea, and uric acid, incorporating the nitrogen into more complex organic molecules. She published this work in the 1902-1903 volume of the *Proceedings of the Royal Society* and concluded, "The effect of this alga, if present, would probably be to leave the water, in which it has grown, in what would be termed a 'more impure' condition."[11]

She had performed careful, scientifically rigorous work. However, the prominent British chemist Henry Roscoe, who studied basic inorganic chemistry and had no interest in public health, reviewed her progress for the 1851 Exhibition Commission. He thought her project in Liverpool was so pedestrian that he recommended against renewing her support and suggested that the sewage commission could pay for the additional year.[12] The 1851 Exhibition Commission nevertheless gave her a second year of funding in the expectation that she would find more interesting work in another laboratory.

Harriette moved to Vienna in 1901 to work with the bacteriologist Max von Gruber. She continued to study dirty water but turned her attention to cleaning it up. She built model sewage treatment plants in the laboratory. Raw liquid sewage, which contains large amounts of ammonia, dripped through cylinders filled with porous coke to which bacteria in the sewage attached. Harriette sampled the effluent from the filters and measured its content of nitrogenous substances.

After the coke-filled cylinders "matured" over a few weeks—that is, gained a stable population of bacteria—the bacteria converted the ammonia to nitrates, which could be concentrated from the efflux and used as agricultural fertilizer. Harriette showed that this process occurred in two stages each requiring a different class of bacteria. She was not ready to write up her results but published an essay pointing out that, although tremendous advances had resulted from Robert Koch's method of obtaining pure cultures of individual species of bacteria, at times, more than one species were required to do the job.[13]

Again, her work was sound but generated little scientific interest. Environmental science had not become a major field of study. The 1851 Exhibition Commission sounded defensive in summing up her performance:

> *Miss Chick's tenure of her Scholarship has been marked by a large amount of useful work in a branch of scientific investigation in which all progress is necessarily very slow. The various investigations have as a rule been conducted with great industry and with adequate skill, and the Scholar has been fortunate in obtaining valuable results.*
>
> *The award of the Scholarship has therefore in this case been amply justified by the character and extent of the work attempted as well as by the importance of the results obtained.*[14]

On returning from Vienna, Harriette moved back in with her parents and two sisters in their house in Ealing and went to work for the Royal Commission on Sewage Disposal. In 1903, she took a leave of absence to complete her studies with Prof. Gruber, who had moved to Munich from Vienna. In addition to scientific training, her time in Vienna and Munich allowed her to perfect her fluency in German, which became important later in her career. After completing her experiments, Harriette published her studies of sewage treatment in in the *Proceedings of the Royal Society*.'[15]

On returning to London and her work for the Royal Commission of Sewage Disposal, she submitted her work with Dr. Boyce on green algae as her doctoral thesis. Once armed with her D.Sc. degree, she secured her position at the Lister Institute and embarked on the career to which she had aspired since high school.

Notes

1   Tomlinson, Margaret (1985) *Three Generations in the Honiton Lace Trade* (Sidmouth, Devon: Sovereign Printing Group), p. 65

2   Sayer, Jane E. (1973) *The Fountain Unsealed. A History of the Notting Hill and Ealing High School.* (Welwyn Garden City, Hertfordshire; Broadwater Press), p. 56.

3   The Completion of the Inner Circle Railway. *The Times of London*, October 7, 1884.

4   Quoted in Sayer, JE (1973) *The Fountain Unsealed*, p. 9.

5   Russell, Bertrand (1967) *The Autobiography of Bertrand Russell, v. 1.* (Boston: Little, Brown), p. 33.

6   Russell, Bertrand, and Russell, Patricia (1937) *The Amberley Papers, v.1.* (New York: Simon and Schuster), p. 17.

7   Tomlinson, M (1983), *Three Generation*, p. 67.

8   Quoted in Sayer, JE (1973) *The Fountain Unsealed*, p. 17.

9   Harte, Negley; North, John; and Brewis, Georgine, eds. (2019) *The World of UCL* (London: UCL Press), p. 51.

10 Jackson, Lee (2014) *Dirty Old London: The Victorian Fight Against Filth.* New Haven: Yale University Press.

11 Chick H (1902-1903) A study of unicellular green algae, occurring in polluted water, with especial reference to its nitrogenous metabolism. *Proc Roy Soc Lond* 71 (467-476): 458-476.

12 Henry Roscoe, note dated 16 June 1900. Archives of the 1851 Exhibition Commission, London.

13 Chick H (1905) The biological limitations of the method of pure culture. *The New Phytologist* 4 (5/6): 120-124.

14 1851 Exhibition Commission (1901) Opinion on the Reports submitted by Miss Harriette Chick, BSC of the University College London, of her work during her tenure for the two years (1899-1901) of a Science Research Scholarship. Archives of the 1851 Exhibition Commission, London.

15 Chick H (1906) A study of the process of nitrification with reference to the purification of sewerage. *Proc Roy Soc Lond* 77 (517): 241-266.

CHAPTER 4
STARTING OUT

In 1905 Harriette went from conducting routine surveillance of London's water to doing original research at the Lister Institute of Preventive Medicine. It had been founded in 1891 to give England a foothold in the burgeoning field of medical science. By the time Harriette joined, it had become the premier medical research facility in Great Britain. Undeterred by the chilly reception by some members of the staff, Harriette Chick devoted her career to that institution. In 1971, in retirement, along with her long-time colleagues Margaret Hume and Marjorie Macfarlane, she published its history in *War on Disease*.[1]

The Lister Institute of Preventive Medicine

In the 1880s the germ theory of disease, pioneered by Louis Pasteur in France, Friedrich Henle and Robert Koch in Germany and Joseph Lister in England, was the most exciting development in the history of medicine. For the first time, scientists were developing effective tools to prevent and treat the world's most common diseases. The advances—smallpox vaccination, pasteurization of milk, diphtheria and tetanus antitoxins—captured the public's attention. Scientists were regularly reporting the discovery of new disease-causing microorganisms and beginning to understand how to harness the immune system to prevent and treat those diseases. The possibilities to improve public health seemed limitless.

England was a leader in the practical application of those discoveries.

The Public Health Act of 1875 divided Great Britain into sanitary districts and provided that each had a Medical Officer of Health. The College of State Medicine was established in 1886 to train those officers. However, England lagged in the basic science. Pasteur had the institute named for him in Paris and Koch had his Institute for Infectious Diseases in Berlin, but there was no similar facility in Great Britain. British scientists who wanted to learn the latest techniques had to travel to the Continent.

The disease that motivated the founding of the Lister Institute was rabies, a disease that the Institute was never to study. Dog ownership in England had grown dramatically during the nineteenth century; and rabies had become a serious problem, especially in the cities where many dogs roamed freely.[2] The bite of a rabid dog injects the virus from its saliva into the victim's blood. After a delay, the virus invades the brainstem and paralyzes the pharyngeal muscles, producing hydrophobia, the inability to swallow. Once neurological symptoms developed, the disease was invariably fatal and was a horrible way to die. In 1885, 672 cases of rabies occurred in England, with 39 deaths in the London area alone. Newspapers described the deaths in gruesome detail, keeping the disease in the public eye.

Louis Pasteur had discovered a method of treating the infection. He injected the rabies virus into rabbits and then dried their spinal cords. He discovered that this process attenuated the virus. That is, the virus lost its ability to cause rabies, but still generated an immune response. A series of injections of an extract of the rabbit spinal cords was lifesaving if begun soon after the dog bite, while the immune system still had a chance to do its job before the virus invaded the brain. The Pasteur Institute generously treated British patients able to travel to Paris.

But the British did not like being dependent on a French institution. In 1889 the Lord Mayor of London convened a committee of doctors, scientists and dog lovers to study the rabies problem. He set in motion discussions of the feasibility of establishing an English counterpart of the Pasteur Institute so that British subjects bitten by rabid dogs did not have to travel to Paris to receive treatment.

The scientists and doctors on the committee strongly supported the proposal. Anti-vivisectionists, a powerful group in Victorian England, opposed it with even greater fervor. That Pasteur killed rabbits to treat rabies was abhorrent to them, and they did not want English rabbits to suffer the same fate. The anti-vivisectionists scored the first victory, flexing their political muscle to persuade the Lord Mayor to disband the committee. However, meeting over tea, some members of the committee formed themselves into an unofficial group to continue to study the feasibility of an English facility modeled on the Pasteur Institute.

Within weeks they issued a report recommending the establishment of a new entity to be called the British Institute of Preventive Medicine. Its mandate would be broader than the treatment of rabies: to study infectious diseases and other aspects of preventive medicine; to produce materials to diagnose, prevent and treat infections; and to train students of public health from any country. To take advantage of existing laboratories and trained staff , the group proposed locating the facility in Cambridge.

The anti-vivisectionists persisted. The Cruelty to Animals Act of 1876 had made animal experimentation a crime without approval from the Home Office. The anti-vivisectionists signed petitions and lobbied to have the approval for the proposed institute denied. The Board of Trade did some political tap dancing. But, prodded by the Prince of Wales and his sister, the Empress Frederick of Germany, the Board of Trade incorporated the Lister Institute on July 25, 1891. The Home Office left the question of permission for animal experimentation unresolved.

The organizers' next task was fundraising, which got off to a slow start. The executors of the estate of an Irishman, Richard Berridge, provided a big boost when they offered £20,000 on the condition that the Institute be located in London. It was an offer the committee could not refuse, especially after the Duke of Westminster offered to sell, at a price substantially less than its market value, land he owned on the Embankment at the Chelsea Bridge. The Berridge estate then donated an additional £25,000. This gave the Committee enough capital to plan and begin building a modern laboratory facility.

They then solved two problems at once by merging with the College of State Medicine. First, the College already had a license to conduct animal experiments and the combined organization could operate under that license. Second, the College had a building at 101 Great Russell Street in Bloomsbury fitted with offices, laboratories, and a library. The British Institute could get started while the new building in Chelsea was under construction. In December 1893, the College of State Medicine merged into the British Institute of Preventive Medicine and came under the direction of a twenty-four member Council.

The anti-vivisectionists did not give up. They went door-to-door throughout Chelsea and collected 183,607 signatures on a petition objecting to the construction of the new building. They claimed, without evidence, that Pasteur was cruel to animals. In addition, they worried that the building would be a health risk to the neighborhood and depress real estate values. The politicians dragged their feet and let construction proceed. In May 1898 the staff of the Institute began to occupy their new laboratories in Chelsea.

Although there was enough money to build the laboratories, the endowment was insufficient to fund ongoing operations. Consequently, in 1898 the Council changed the name from the British Institute to the Jenner Institute of Preventive Medicine to honor Edward Jenner, the English country physician who, a hundred years earlier, had inoculated a boy with cowpox and prevented his death from smallpox.

Jenner's name was recognized throughout the world and the Council hoped that patriotic pride would pry open the British purses. The strategy failed; the public contributed only £70. Edward Guinness—Lord Iveagh, the owner of the Guinness brewery—donated £5,000, not sufficient to endow the Jenner Institute of Preventive Medicine but enough to fund the Jenner Memorial Research Studentship, which later supported Harriette Chick during her first two years at the Institute.

Rabies again played a role when a case prompted Lord Iveagh to become the Institute's major benefactor. In 1898, a rabid dog bit one of his long-term employees. The man received treatment at the Pasteur Institute and suffered no long-term effects. Lord Iveagh visited the Pasteur Institute and was impressed. He was already planning a large gift to promote a worthy cause in London and decided to direct £250,000 to the Jenner Institute on the condition that there be a change in governance to give him more control. It was another offer the Council could not refuse. A new entity, the Governing Body, took over responsibility for the policies and finances of the Institute and the

Council demoted itself to an advisory capacity. Of the seven members of the Governing Body, Lord Iveagh appointed three, the Council of the Institute appointed three and the Royal Society one. This system survived, with minor tweaks, for the life of the Institute.

Not only did the name change to the Jenner Institute not attract a flood of donations, it provoked a legal battle with the owner of a private business called The Jenner Institute for Calf Lymph, which sold the smallpox vaccine invented by Jenner. Rather than prolong the conflict, in 1903 the Council relented and adopted the name Lister Institute for Preventive Medicine, honoring Joseph Lister, the proponent of surgical disinfection and first president of the Governing Body.

When Harriette arrived at the Lister Institute, the brick and stone building at the Chelsea Bridge was state-of-the-art. "Bright, spacious and lofty laboratories, with teak work-benches and pine-block floors, were equipped with the most up-to-date apparatus of the day."[3] The five-story structure housed four stories of laboratories and offices. The top floor contained the Director's residence and a library. The basement housed a workshop for fashioning and repairing laboratory apparatus, a warm room to culture bacteria, a refrigerated room to store supplies, and a room dedicated to the preparation of culture media. The building even had central heating, a rare luxury for turn-of-the-century London.

Fourteen staff scientists, six guest workers and about twelve laboratory technicians staffed the laboratories when they opened. Most of the scientists studied infectious disease, but others studied nutrition, cellular metabolism and cancer. The laboratories were not segregated by discipline and the scientists mingled freely. The staff, especially the guest workers, expanded quickly and another wing was added to the original structure. Once up and running, with no disaster befalling Chelsea, the neighborhood opposition dissipated.

According to Harriette, "The Institute became a kind of club, rigid in standards, informal in manner; a little puzzling to strangers, remembered nostalgically by its guests, held in pride and an often exasperated affection by its more permanent residents." To its scientific staff "the Institute was not merely a place where they were employed but a way of life, a habit of thought."[4] It became the focus of Harriette's life.

A New Job and a New Boss

Harriette began her career at the Lister Institute at the age of thirty supported by the Jenner Memorial Research Studentship. She never wrote about what she experienced as the first woman to break the gender barrier. Later in life, she made light of the sexism she had faced. However, she was not completely passive, as she advocated for women's suffrage. In 1914, she is listed as a co-signer of a letter to a weekly newspaper, *Votes for Women*, protesting the decision of the Prime Minister and Parliament to table the issue of enfranchising women.[5] She signed the letter as Secretary of the Women's Suffrage Committee of the London Graduates Union.

In Dr. Martin's laboratory she functioned as a postdoctoral fellow. Under his mentorship she thrived. As she later wrote, "Martin had a gift for discovering special talents in his staff and could encourage their development without interfering with their freedom."[6] She became the prime example of Martin's gift. They rapidly bonded and he became her close friend as well as her mentor.

Charles James Martin was born in the outskirts of London in 1866. Harriette quotes him as saying, "the family into which I was born was a Nonconformist middle-class one characteristic of the period, with lots of children, a fading flavour of piety and a small revenue."[7] His father was an insurance actuary and hoped that Charles would follow in his footsteps. At the age of fifteen, after graduation from secondary school, Charles had to earn his keep and took a job as a junior clerk in the same insurance company for which his father worked. To prepare himself for a career as an actuary, he took courses in mathematics. He was not especially good at it and began to study chemistry.

Over the objections of his family, he aspired to become a doctor. They agreed that if he passed the entrance examination for medical school, he could pursue that career. He took evening classes, including chemistry, at Birbeck College and King's College. He bought a used copy of *A Hundred Experiments in Chemistry* and compulsively went through all hundred experiments in an outhouse of his family's residence. At age 17 he passed the entrance examination for the University of London and his family acquiesced to his becoming a medical student at St. Thomas Hospital.

There, he befriended F. Gowland Hopkins, who at the time was an analytical chemist at the hospital and allowed Martin to perform experiments in his laboratory. Martin claimed partial credit for convincing Hopkins, the future Nobel Prize winner, to give up his career as a chemist and study medicine. After earning a B.Sc. degree with honors from the University of London, Martin first went to Leipzig to study physiology with Carl Ludwig. Following that, he held a teaching post at King's College, his day job, while he continued to study medicine at St. Thomas Hospital in his free time, earning his medical degree in 1890.

Nothing in Martin's life to this point was unusual for an intelligent and ambitious middle-class young man of his times. His leadership skills only came to light when he moved to Australia in 1891 to take up teaching posts. The salaries of junior faculty were substantially better in Australia than England and he had a new bride and soon a daughter to support. He stayed for twelve years, working first at the University of Sydney and then in Melbourne. He made a big impact on Australian medicine and on his students; they spoke of "the Martin spirit." He studied the mechanism of action of snake venoms and, based on that work, was elected Fellow of the Royal Society in 1901. In 1903 he came back to England to take over as Director of the Lister Institute, where he remained until he nominally retired in 1930.

All commentators speak of his intelligence, breadth of knowledge, and phenomenal memory. They also speak of his modesty and ability to provide both wise guidance and independence to his colleagues. When he took over as Director of the Institute, it was twelve years old and had a spotty record of scientific productivity. Under his leadership it rapidly became the major medical research facility in Great Britain, a status it maintained through the end of World War I.

The Science of Disinfectants

Harriette Chick started in Martin's laboratory studying disinfection. When Pasteur and Koch discovered that microorganisms caused disease, the search immediately began for ways to kill the potentially deadly microbes. Antibiotics were decades in the future and researchers were only beginning to understand bacterial biology. The only way to kill the germs was by brute force: subjecting them to high temperatures or flooding them with poisons, termed *disinfectants*. Among the most effective disinfectants were phenols (contained in coal tar and also known as carbolic acid) and certain metal salts, including mercuric chloride and silver nitrate. However, as Harriette wrote, "In the young science of bacteriology the principles underlying the process of disinfection were not understood and there was no reliable technique for testing the claims made for the efficacy of disinfectants."[8]

From the point of view of the twenty-first century, the study of these crude methods seems uninteresting; but in 1905 it was cutting edge science with practical value. Joseph Lister had shown that disinfection in the operating room and the maternity ward profoundly reduced deaths from infections. Although there were no antibiotics, physicians used antisera to neutralize diphtheria and tetanus toxins. Maintaining the sterility of the sera during their preparation and storage were essential to their safe use. On a larger scale, efficient methods to disinfect sewerage before being discharged into the Thames might protect London from water-borne infectious diseases.

There were two popular theories to explain how disinfectants killed bacteria. One was *vitalism*, which held that all living things, including bacteria, possessed an ill-defined "life force" and that disinfectants poisoned that life force. The strength of the life force in a population of bacteria was assumed to follow a bell-shaped curve. Vitalism therefore predicted that after the application of a disinfectant the rate of death of bacteria, measured as the number of bacteria dying per unit of time, would follow a similar bell curve. The rate of death would start slowly as the minority with a weak life force died. The large majority in the middle would die next and, because of their numbers, at a rapid rate. The minority with the strongest life force would die the slowest.

Harriette held to the alternative, *mechanistic*, school of thought. She believed that disinfection was a chemical reaction between the disinfectant and some component of the bacteria. If she were correct, disinfection would follow the laws of an ordinary chemical reaction in which the rate of the reaction depends on the concentration of reagents. In the case of a culture of bacteria exposed to a disinfectant, the rate of death would be greatest immediately after the application of the disinfectant when the concentration of living bacteria was greatest.

While trying to discover how disinfectants killed germs, her first job was to perfect and standardize the experimental methods so that laboratories could compare results. Previous workers had evolved a simple experimental design. A culture of a single bacterial species was prepared in liquid broth providing all the required nutrients. To test a disinfectant, a small amount of the bacterial culture was transferred to another tube containing the disinfectant. As the bacteria sat in the disinfectant, samples were removed at various times and mixed with liquid agar, which was allowed to gel, fixing each bacterium in place. After culturing in agar for 24-48 hours, each individual bacterium reproduced many times and formed a visible colony, allowing the number of colonies, hence the number of bacteria that survived the disinfectant, to be counted.

For her initial paper, published in 1908, she used anthrax spores and paratyphoid bacteria to perfect the experimental methodology.[9] She first had to solve seemingly trivial problems, such as how to best transfer the bacteria from one vessel to another. Whereas previous workers had used threads or tiny garnets, Harriette used pipettes to quantify the amount transferred more precisely. But the bacteria stuck to the pipette tips and she had to demonstrate that her pipettes were identical and reliably transferred the same number of bacteria. She next had to deal with the small amount of disinfectant carried over into the final culture in agar. It turned out not to be a problem for relatively weak disinfectants, such as phenols; but metallic salts were so potent that she had to develop methods to precipitate them out of solution before adding the bacteria to the agar.

After resolving the methodological issues, she studied the time course of disinfection and modeled it mathematically. She found that the rate of killing was maximal immediately after applying the disinfectant and gradually slowed, following the time course of a first-order chemical reaction. That is, the rate of killing was proportional to the number of remaining living bacteria. She also showed that the influence of temperature followed the laws of chemical reactions. In sum, "A very complete analogy exists between a chemical reaction and the process of disinfection, one reagent being represented by the disinfectant, and the second by the protoplasm of the bacterium."

Harriette came down firmly on the side of the mechanistic explanation. Her application of quantitative methods to answer biological questions was innovative at the time. As Harriette wrote, "There was strong criticism of a mechanistic attitude which likened the behavior of a biological entity, the living bacterial cell, to that of non-living substances involved in chemical reactions."[10] The scientific revolution was not yet complete.

A Month in Germany

We have few views into Harriette's inner life, but some of her diaries have survived. Most entries are records of the weather, work meetings and meals. However, one record is more intimate, a journal of a month of walking in Germany in 1906.[11] She traveled with her sisters Elsie and Edith and two men, Arthur and Eric, whose relationship to the women is not described. They left on August 9. Harriette began the journey depressed because of "a variety of circumstances at home" and noted that "we always go abroad depressed." She became even more depressed when she saw the cramped accommodations on board the ship they were taking to Germany.

Her record of the first days in Germany continues in this negative vein, mainly concerned with sore feet and missed train connections. Once they arrived in Bayreuth, however, the tone changes. Harriette was a music lover and attending concerts was one of her favorite ways to relax. She wrote about the opera and symphony concerts they attended, giving them mixed reviews. She described the meals they enjoyed, the sights they admired, and the friends they met along the way. "The country is a Durer etching land," she wrote. She recorded the events of each day but did not write about the interpersonal relationships among her companions.

In an event reminiscent of E. M. Forster's novel *Howard's End*, Arthur lost his umbrella at a concert. Harriette took up the search. "I think we had become imbued with the romantic spirit;" "...the spirit of the chase was in my blood." The umbrella was recovered the next day. However, unlike the novel, in Harriette's diary the recovery of the lost umbrella does not lead to a romance.

Toward the end of the trip, on September 4, Elsie became ill. Edith, Eric, and Arthur departed for home, leaving Harriette to care for the invalid. She does not note why she was given this responsibility or how she felt about it, but it was consistent with her sense of duty. Elsie rapidly recovered and the two of them, with a Mr. Blackburn, rode a coach to board a boat down the Rhine. Harriette arrived back at the family home in Ealing on September 8, exactly a month after leaving.

The Chick-Martin Test

Back in the laboratory, after her studies on the mechanism of action of disinfectants, Harriette worked on a method to compare them quantitatively.[12] Previously, Samuel Rideal and J. T. Ainslie Walker had developed a method to compare a test agent with phenol, producing a *carbolic acid (or phenol) coefficient* expressing the strength of the test substance relative to phenol dissolved in distilled water. Harriette thought that their method did not represent real-world conditions, since disinfectants typically were not used in clean water but wiped on dirty surfaces or added to filthy sewage. Also, the Rideal-Walker method did not specify a fixed time for the reaction; different phenol coefficients could be obtained for a disinfectant depending on how long the reaction was carried out.

Harriette modified the Rideal-Walker method by specifying that the reaction proceed for 30 minutes and by adding dried human feces to the disinfectant solutions. Her test, called the *Chick-Martin test*, with minor modifications, was used into the 1960s. It has since been superseded by tests to determine the optimum concentration of disinfectants for specific purposes.[13]

She published two more papers dealing with disinfection. One explained the superiority of emulsified over soluble disinfectants by their adsorption to the surface of the bacteria, thereby increasing their effective concentration.[14] The final paper described disinfection by hot water, once again showing the process obeyed known principles of chemical reactions and laying the foundation for her later studies of protein denaturation by heat.[15]

Harriette wrote her early papers in a style typical for the times and much different from that of twenty-first century scientific communications. They are long—one is over sixty pages—and describe the methodology in meticulous detail, recounting her thought processes along the way. Continuing her innovative approach, she fit her data to mathematical models whenever she could. As time went on, her writing style conformed to the standards of the day, but she always described her methods with great care.

The Coagulation of Proteins

Harriette's studies of disinfectants convinced her that they killed bacteria by reacting chemically with the bacterial protoplasm. At the turn of the twentieth century, before the role of nucleic acids was understood, biologists thought that proteins were the key components of life. Harriette naturally assumed that her disinfectants were reacting with bacterial proteins. Therefore, she next turned her attention to fundamental biochemistry, studying how proteins denature, that is, how they lose their shape and their biological activity.

She studied the heat-induced coagulation of proteins as a model of denaturation. The coagulation of egg white in a boiled egg is an example of that process. Harriette heated hemoglobin or egg albumin in a water bath and measured the rate at which the protein coagulated into clumps that would not pass through filter paper. She found that coagulation occurred in two stages: first, heat forces water into the protein molecule causing it to swell and denature; then, the individual protein molecules clump together to form the coagulate. The second step was so fast that, in practice, she was measuring the rate of the first stage.

She found that the coagulation of hemoglobin closely followed the time course of a simple chemical reaction. The behavior of albumin was more complicated, due to gains and losses of ions as the protein lost its compact shape. She therefore carried out detailed investigations of the effects of acids, bases and salts on the process. With a constant ionic composition and pH of the solvent, albumin followed the same rules as hemoglobin. She and Martin published the findings in a series of four papers in the *Journal of Physiology*, fleshing out their mechanistic view of disinfection.[16]

Chick next turned her attention to serum. She published a study of the ability of rabbit serum to kill E. coli, but this line of investigation led nowhere.[17] She next carried out a productive series of experiments on serum proteins. The antisera given to people to neutralize bacterial toxins were prepared by immunizing animals, usually horses. Horses too old and decrepit to continue pulling carts were readily available and they produce much more serum than small laboratory animals such as rabbits. Although the immune system remained a mystery, it was known that a type of protein called an antibody was the component of serum that neutralized the toxins.

Biochemists divided serum proteins into classes based on their solubility properties and separated them by a process termed *salting out*. By gradually adding ammonium sulfate to serum, a class of protein called *euglobulins* first precipitates out of solution. At a higher concentration of ammonium sulfate, another class called *pseudoglobulins* precipitates. The albumin is the last to come out of solution. This process was of practical use. The pseudoglobulin fraction contains the antibodies, which can be concentrated by salting out, producing a more potent antiserum and minimizing the exposure of patients to foreign proteins.

Salting out works because the salt competes with the protein for water molecules that keep the protein in solution. Harriette quantified the potency of different salts and the effects of acid-base balance on the process. She and Martin published these results in the *Biochemical Journal*, the major journal in the field at that time.[18]

Collectively these papers, along with her studies of disinfectants and protein coagulation, established Harriette Chick as a mature and independent scientist. Moreover, it solidified her relationship with her mentor and champion, Charles Martin, the Boss. This was a solid foundation for a career in basic biochemistry. In 1913 she became one of the first three women admitted to membership in the Biochemical Society, which a year earlier had changed its name from the Biochemical Club and changed its by-laws to allow *persons* to be members rather than only *men*.[19] She might well have gone on to make major discoveries in bacterial metabolism or protein chemistry, but World War I put an abrupt end to that line of work.

The Demands of War

With the outbreak of World War I in August 1914, everything changed at the Institute. Almost all the men left to join the military and the women took over the laboratory work[20]. Moreover, the nature of that work shifted dramatically. The Lister Institute had two main purposes: first, to do basic scientific research related to public health and, second, "to prepare and supply special protective and curative materials, such as vaccines and antitoxins." The war pushed the first purpose onto the back burner.

The troops were endangered not only by enemy guns and artillery but also from wound infections and contagious diseases spread in the crowded and unsanitary trenches. Martin was especially concerned that in the manure-fertilized fields in France, tetanus would be a major threat. He wanted to ensure that the Institute could supply the army with sufficient tetanus antitoxin and crucial diagnostic and therapeutic sera. He closed his laboratory and focused on organizing the women at the Lister to carry out this work.

Martin did not enjoy this purely administrative work. He developed a flu-like illness compounded by stress. Harriette became so concerned about his health that she went to Sir Henry Roscoe, Chairman of the Governing Body. On May 14, 1915, Roscoe wrote to Harriette:

> I am sure that you will have been pleased to learn that acting upon the conversation you and I had as to Martin's health the GB [Governing Body], without consultation with him, decided that he is to have leave of absence for two months. You were the first person to place the case before me and I at once obtained Mr. Pattisson's [the Treasurer] acquiescence and afterwards the unanimous decision of the GB.
>
> I was glad to learn that Martin had expressed himself relieved that the responsibility of taking a holiday was removed from his shoulders. The sooner he can get away the better.[21]

Martin asked Harriette Chick to take over the production of tetanus antiserum. Like other antisera, it was prepared in horses. To house the animals and the preparative work, the institute had bought a farm in Elstree, a suburb about fifteen miles north of central London. The tetanus work was so dangerous that it had its own building. Harriette and her assistants, other women transferred from Chelsea, prepared cultures of the bacterium, *Clostridium tetani*, and extracted and purified the lethal toxin. They injected escalating doses of the toxin into horses until the animals became immune. If they increased the dose too rapidly, they killed the horse. When a horse was fully immunized, they bled it and prepared the globulin containing the anti-tetanus antibody. All the while, they had to maintain sterility and ensure that the antitoxin was safe to inject into humans.

Harriette did not enjoy her new assignment. The dangerous and exacting work was crucial to the war effort, but it was uninteresting. Plus, the commute was onerous. To get to Elstree from Ealing, she had to take two trains and walk from the station, a walk that wound through well-kempt rural fields but was unpleasant in bad weather. Once she arrived, she had to work in a poorly heated building.

The worst aspect of the assignment was that the director of the serum department in Elstree, Dr. Alfred MacConkey, was a "natural dictator with some peculiar traits, and not an easy colleague."[22] Harriette and her colleagues, accustomed to the freedom and collegial atmosphere in Chelsea, found the environment in Elstree intolerable and complained to Dr. Martin. MacConkey responded by dispatching the uppity women back to Chelsea.

Happily back in more comfortable surroundings, Harriette took on equally routine but less dangerous work preparing antisera to diagnose typhoid, paratyphoid and dysentery. She expected to continue this task indefinitely when she received a message from Dr. Martin, by this time Lt. Col. Martin, asking her to change direction once again.

A Message from Lemnos

Dr. Martin extended his leave of absence by enlisting in the military. Although English by birth, he joined the Australian Army Medical Corps, having lived in Australia for twelve years. He was assigned to serve as a pathologist for the No. 3 Australian General Hospital in Mudos on the Greek island of Lemnos. The island served as the primary evacuation site for the soldiers of the Australian and New Zealand Army Corps (ANZAC), a major component of the amphibious landing of Entente forces on the Gallipoli Peninsula on April 25, 1915.

The Gallipoli campaign was a military disaster and was eventually abandoned in December 1916 after 250,000 casualties, including at least 50,000 deaths. The hospital facilities on Lemnos grew to 10,000 beds to accommodate the flood of sick and wounded soldiers. Martin had to build and maintain a pathology laboratory, mainly housed in tents subject to being blown over by winds of up to 70 miles per hour.

Martin wrote frequent letters back to England describing his daily life and his challenges. Many of his letters were saved by his daughter Maisie and published by her son Martin Gibbs in a self-published biography of his grandfather.[23] Harriette Chick, H. C. as he addressed her in his letters, was his second most frequent correspondent after Maisie. He later wrote to Harriette:

You are the most interesting correspondent I have encountered. I have all of your letters filed and when you're dead I propose to make my fortune by publishing them at popular prices.[24]

Unfortunately, Harriette's letters to the Boss have been lost.

Martin's letters had to pass the censors and mainly dealt with mundane matters and giving thanks for gifts of warm clothing, including a pair of socks and a balaclava from Harriette. In November 1914 there was an exchange of letters addressing whether Harriette should join Martin on Lemnos. He wrote to her:

Now to the question of your joining us and seeing life. The reason I have said nothing previously was the extraordinary uncertainty of everything in this part of the world. At any moment we might be shifted elsewhere. I was naturally averse to your being attached to some unit and I to another where we should not work together.

I have made inquiries and the only chance of your coming here is to take a job as nursing sister in the Australian army, earmarked by arrangement for laboratory duty. Sex discipline has to be severe on active service, quite apart from the ancient prejudices of the powers. The sisters are absolutely under the discipline of the matron in everything outside their professional work. I don't know whether you would

like such a position but if you would I might be able to get it arranged
with the Australians.

Let me know your views. Meantime I will open negotiations and
if nothing comes of it no harm will be done. I need hardly say that it
would be a great joy to me if you came but I hardly think you will make
the necessary sacrifice of your individual freedom.[25]

In the end, the authorities did not approve Harriette's move. Furthermore, as Harriette wrote, "We both realized that I was more useful maintaining a base at the Lister Institute and carrying on special research there."[26]

When Martin arrived on Lemnos in the summer of 1915, he found some soldiers suffering from degeneration of the nerves in their legs. The condition had baffled the hospital's doctors; but Martin recognized it as *tropical beriberi,* a disease that he had learned about from investigators in his department at the Lister Institute.

Beriberi had become endemic in Asia during the nineteenth century when white rice replaced brown rice as the dietary staple. The white rice lacked an essential nutrient, now known to be thiamin (vitamin B1). Two Lister Institute scientists, Casimir Funk and Evelyn Ashley Cooper, had studied the disease in guinea pigs and tried, unsuccessfully, to identify the missing substance.

The troops at Gallipoli had been living on tinned meat and jam spread on bread and biscuits made from white flour. Dr. Martin surmised that white flour lacked the same unknown substance as white rice. He believed the Lister Institute could help solve the problem and find a way to prevent the disease. But, after the war broke out, Casimir Funk moved to the United States and Evelyn Ashley Cooper joined the army. Therefore, Charles Martin sent a message to Harriette asking her to turn over serum production to others and devote her efforts to determining what foods the army could give the troops to prevent beriberi.

Harriette welcomed the change and was eager to assemble a team and get started on the new project. It would support the troops and at the same time allow her to make new discoveries. What she did not realize was that this was a permanent change in her career. It would establish her as a leader of British science, help catalyze the growth of nutrition research worldwide, and lead her to make a major impact on public health.

Notes

1   Chick, Harriette; Hume, Margaret; and Macfarlane, Margorie (1971) *War on Disease. A History of the Lister Institute.* London: Andre Deutsch.

2   Walton, JK (1979) Mad dogs and Englishmen: the conflict over rabies in late Victorian England. *J Social History* 13: 219-239.

3   Chick H et al. (1971) *War on Disease*, p. 54.

4   Chick H et al. (1971) *War on Disease*, p. 14.

5   Gwynne-Vaughan HCJ, Roberts AM, Busk M, Chick H (June 19, 1914) The Plural Voting Bill. *Votes for Women* VII (328): 578.

6   Chick H et al. (1971) *War on Disease*, p. 71.

7   Chick H (1956) Charles James Martin. 1866-1955. *Biographical Memoirs of Fellows of the Royal Society* 2: 172-208.

8   Chick H et al. (1971) *War on Disease*, p. 87.

9   Chick H (1908) An investigation of the laws of disinfection. *J Hygiene (Lond)* 8 (1): 92-158.

10   Chick H et al. *War on Disease*, p.91.

11   Chick H (1906), personal diary, Wellcome Library, London.

12   Chick H, Martin CJ (1908a) The principle involved in the standardization of disinfectants and the influence or organic matter upon germicidal value. *J Hyg (Lond)* 8 (5): 654-697.

13   Baxby D (1908) The Chick-Martin test for disinfectants. *Epidemiol Infect* 133 (Suppl. 1) S13-S14.

14   Chick H, Martin CJ (1908b) A comparison of the power of a germicide emulsified or dissolved, with an interpretation of the superiority of the emulsified form. *J Hyg (Lond)* 8 (5): 698-703.

15   Chick H (1910) The process of disinfection by chemical agencies and hot water. *J Hyg (Lond)* 10 (2): 237-286.

16   Chick H, Martin CJ (1910) On the "heat coagulation" of proteins. *J Physiol* 40 (5): 404 – 430.

Chick H, Martin CJ (1911) On the "heat coagulation" of proteins. Part II. The action of hot water upon egg-albumen and the influence of acid and salts upon reaction velocity. *J Physiol* 43 (1): 1 – 27.

Chick H, Martin CJ (1912) On the "heat coagulation" of proteins. Part III. The influence of alkali upon reaction velocity. *J Physiol* 45 (1-2): 61-69.

Chick H, Martin CJ (1912) On the "heat coagulation" of proteins. Part IV. The conditions controlling the agglutination of proteins already acted upon by hot water. *J Physiol* 45 (4): 261 – 295.

17   Chick H (1912) The bactericidal properties of blood serum. I. The reaction-velocity of the germicidal action of normal rabbit-serum on *B. coli commue* and the influence of temperature thereon. *J Hyg (Lond)* 12 (4): 414-435.

18   Chick H, Martin CJ (1913) The density and solution volume of some proteins. *Biochem J* 7 (1): 92-96.

Chick H (1913) The factors concerned in the solution and precipitation of euglobulin. *Biochem J* 7 (3): 318-340.

Chick H, Martin CJ (1913) The precipitation of egg-albumin by ammonium sulfate. A contribution to the theory of the "salting-out" of proteins. *Biochem J* 7 (4): 380-398.

Chick H, Lubrzynska E (1914) The viscosity of some protein solutions. *Biochem J* 8 (1): 59-69.

Chick H (1914) The viscosity of protein solutions. II. Pseudoglobulin and euglobulin (horse). *Biochem J* 8 (3): 261-280.

Chick H (1914) The apparent formation of euglobulin from pseudo-globulin and a suggestion as to the relationship between these two proteins in serum. *Biochem J* 8 (4):404-420.

19   *Women in the Biochemical Society* (10 November 2010) Centre for the History of Medicine, University of Warwick. https://warwick.ac.uk/fac/arts/history/chm/research/womenbiochemists/biochemicalsociety

20   Fara, Patricia. (2018) *A Lab of One's Own. Science and Suffrage in the First World War.* Oxford: Oxford University Press.

21   Gibbs, Martin (2011) *Charles Martin. His Life and Letters.* (London: Martin Gibbs), p. 84.

22   Chick H et al. (1971) *War on Disease*, p. 82

23   Gibbs Martin (2011) *Charles Martin. His Life and Letters.* London: Martin Gibbs.

24   Gibbs M (2011) *Charles Martin,* p. 104.

25   Gibbs M (2011) *Charles Martin,* p. 95.

26   Gibbs M (2011) *Charles Martin,* p.101.

CHAPTER 5

NUTRITION AS SCIENCE

When Harriette Chick entered nutrition research, the field was a century old and had grown into an important branch of physiology. However, the study of vitamins was still in its infancy; and vitamin deficiency diseases, which had killed millions over the past four centuries, remained a threat to public health.

Beriberi (thiamin, or vitamin B1, deficiency) was a major killer in Asia. Scurvy (vitamin C deficiency) had ceased to be a scourge of sailors but still afflicted polar explorers, soldiers with stretched supply lines, and infants who were fed artificial formulas rather than breast milk or whose nursing mothers were malnourished. Rickets (vitamin D deficiency) stunted the growth and deformed the limbs of children in industrial cities across Europe and North America. And pellagra (niacin, or vitamin B3, deficiency) was rife in areas of Europe and North America where the poor depended on corn and cornmeal for most of their food.

It took almost four centuries to recognize that vitamin deficiency diseases even existed. The journal of the first voyage of Vasco da Gama, written during the final years of the fifteenth century, described scurvy decimating the crew as they sailed up the east coast of Africa. The journal also noted that when the men ate oranges, they rapidly recovered. However, the concept that one could consume sufficient calories but still have a nutritional deficiency was alien; and other mechanisms were invoked to explain the benefit of citrus fruit.

Diseases were ascribed to outside agents such as infections, bad air or toxins. It was not until the early nineteenth century that nutrition began to be studied in animals, allowing rigorous scientific experimentation. The first efforts were in France.

Feeding the Poor

The laboratory investigation of nutrition began in 1815 with the formation of the Gelatin Commission in Paris.[1] Led by the noted physiologist Francois Magendie, the Commission started with the belief that animals, including humans, required only a source of energy—either carbohydrates or fat—plus protein to survive. They intended to show that people, specifically the growing population of urban poor, could live on a diet limited to bread as a source of energy and gelatin* as a source of protein.

The Gelatin Commission failed in that attempt but introduced two key innovations: the use of animal models in nutrition research and the study of simplified diets. Magendie used dogs in his experiments, assuming that the nutritional requirements of all mammals, including humans, were similar. He fed the dogs simple, well-defined diets, such as sugar alone, bread alone or both bread and gelatin. The dogs could not remain healthy more than a few weeks on these diets, but the reductionist strategy of feeding purified nutrients became fundamental to nutrition research.

During the second half of the nineteenth century, nutrition scientists exploited discoveries in chemistry, coming mainly from laboratories in Germany, to build on the work of the Gelatin Commission. They focused on two questions: the energy content of foods, measured in calories, and the nutritional quality of purified proteins. The study of the first of these questions defined the caloric needs of people of various sizes and activity levels and determined how much of which nutrients would satisfy those needs.

The second question sprang from the recognition that all proteins were not equally nutritious. If restricted to zein, the main protein in maize, as its only source of protein, a rat would lose weight and die. But, casein, the major milk protein, could support its survival as long as other essential nutrients

---

* Gelatin is primarily composed of the protein collagen, which is extracted by boiling animal connective tissues.

were provided. The new methods of chemical analysis demonstrated that proteins were composed of up to twenty different amino acids and that proteins differed in their content of those constituents. Zein for example, lacked the essential amino acid tryptophan. Scientists spent great effort in comparing the nutritional properties of purified proteins.

This line of research progressed in a straightforward manner, beginning with the Gelatin Commission and continuing through the first decades of the twentieth century. The discovery of vitamins took a more circuitous route, requiring that investigators abandon common wisdom and explore unexpected findings.

A Medical Student is Ignored

The first experimental evidence of the requirement for micronutrients came in 1881 from a Russian medical student, Nicolai Lunin, working in the laboratory of the prominent physiologist Gustav von Bunge in Basel, Switzerland.[2] When Lunin fed his mice cow's milk, they remained healthy. Lunin's innovation was to separate the milk into its major ingredients: casein, milk fat, lactose (the main sugar in milk), and inorganic salts. When he mixed these ingredients back together and fed the mixture to his mice, they died within weeks even though they obtained sufficient calories. He concluded that milk contains a small amount of some nutrient essential to life, something he had lost in the process of purifying milk's individual constituents.

Von Bunge dismissed his student's conclusion. He was convinced that all that was required for a healthy diet was energy from carbohydrates and fats, the necessary proteins, and inorganic salts. His own research focused on the inorganic substances and he thought that in separating the milk into its components, Lunin had converted some inorganic molecule into an inactive form.

Although other students of von Bunge repeated Lunin's findings, no one tried to find the missing nutrient. Accepting von Bunge's views, scientists ignored the work of the Russian medical student for two decades. Nevertheless, talent won out and Lunin prospered. He gave up vitamin research after leaving von Bunge's laboratory; but he completed clinical training in Western

Europe, returned to Russia, and enjoyed a distinguished career as a pediatrician in St. Petersburg.[3]

A Giant Step

The next breakthrough on the path to the discovery of vitamins came not from a modern university chemistry laboratory but from a bare-bones facility attached to a military hospital in the outskirts of Djakarta on the Indonesian island of Java.[4]

In 1886 the Dutch government dispatched the physician Christiaan Eijkman to Java to find the microbe causing the epidemic of beriberi in Asia.[*] The disease ravaged Southeast Asia and Japan during the nineteenth century, when the invention of the steam-driven milling machine made white rice cheap enough to replace brown rice as a staple of the diet. In addition to causing degeneration of the peripheral nerves, with numbness, weakness, and muscle wasting, beriberi went on to kill by causing heart failure. Beriberi came to rival infections as the major cause of death in Southeast Asia.

A grain of rice consists of three layers: an outer, indigestible husk; underlying layers of reddish-brown cells that form the *silverskin* (also called the *bran* or *pericarp*); and the white core (*endocarp*) consisting almost entirely of starch. At the base of each grain is the germ, the actual seed. Prior to the invention of mechanical milling machines, the husks were removed by pounding the grains with a pestle followed by winnowing to separate the husks, leaving brown rice, the core covered by the silverskin and retaining the germ. White rice required further polishing by hand to remove the silverskin and germ, a time-consuming process making white rice too expensive for all but the wealthy.

The mechanical milling machine made the process cheap enough to allow the masses to afford white rice, which was generally preferred over brown. However, the thiamin is mainly contained in the germ and pericarp. Thus, the common Asian diet of that time—white rice and some fish or meat, with little fresh fruit or vegetables—provided virtually no thiamin.

At the end of the nineteenth century, none of this was understood. The

---

* The origin of the word *beriberi* is not known for certain. It may have arisen from a Sinhalese phrase meaning "weak, weak." In Japan, the disease was called *kakke*.

germ theory dominated medical thinking; and physicians speculated that beriberi was an infection, perhaps caused by a microbe that produced a neurotoxin. Christiaan Eijkman was the perfect man to test this theory, having worked in Robert Koch's bacteriology laboratory. He started out using rabbits for his experiments but switched to chickens, which were cheaper. He injected one group of chickens with the blood of patients hospitalized with beriberi. Chickens in the control group were not injected. He predicted that the patients' blood would transfer the microbe, and the disease, to the injected chickens and his control chickens would remain healthy.

At first, nothing happened and Eijkman made no progress. But suddenly, in July 1889, all his chickens, whether or not they had been injected with patients' blood, began losing weight and developing leg weakness. When examined pathologically, they had the same pattern of nerve degeneration as people with beriberi. He called this disease *polyneuritis gallinarum* (inflammation of chicken nerves), but it was the avian form of beriberi. His use of chickens for his experiments was fortuitous, as birds develop the signs of thiamin deficiency before other vitamin deficiencies become manifest.

Still adhering to the germ theory, Eijkman hypothesized that the chickens caught the disease through the air, explaining why even the group that was not injected with patients' blood got the disease. He began experiments to test his hypothesis and soon got another surprise. In November, as suddenly as all his chickens had started getting sick, they stopped developing the disease.

Eijkman learned that the man taking care of his chickens had made a change in their diet just before they began developing leg weakness. Originally, he fed the chickens whole-grain rice, the cheapest form. Chickens grind off the indigestible husks in their gizzards, leaving what is essentially brown rice to digest. However, Eijkman's conscientious helper wanted to economize even more and persuaded the hospital cook to donate the patients' leftover white rice to the chickens. Within weeks, the chickens began to develop beriberi. But when a new cook arrived in November, in Eijkman's words, he "refused to allow military rice to be taken for civilian chickens."[5] When the chickens returned to eating whole-grain rice, they remained healthy.

Eijkman repeated the serendipitous experiment. When he fed chickens whole-grain rice or brown rice, they did fine. When he fed them white rice, they developed leg weakness. When he gave them back rice bran, or an aqueous extract of the bran, along with the white rice, the chickens remained strong. Still unwilling to abandon the germ theory, he speculated that the rice core was infected with a neurotoxin-producing microbe—or perhaps rice starch contained a substance that was converted into a toxin by bacteria in the intestine—and the bran contained an antidote.

In 1896, Eijkman became ill from malaria and had to return to Holland. Gerrit Grijns, a physician with a background in physiology rather than bacteriology, came to Java to take over the work. He repeated Eijkman's rice experiments, with the same results. He also showed that other carbohydrate-rich diets, such as potato flour and milk sugar, produced the same pattern of nerve degeneration as white rice, making the infected rice theory highly unlikely. He also found that feeding legumes, such as certain beans or peas, along with white rice prevented the disease.

Grijns became friendly with another Dutch physician, Adolphe Vorderman, who had worked in Indonesia for twenty years and was the medical inspector of the prisons on the island of Java, which housed almost a quarter of a million prisoners. He knew that the incidence of beriberi varied widely among the prisons and that the prisons prepared their rice differently. He surveyed the prisons and found that beriberi was much more common in those serving white rice than those using brown rice, reinforcing the results of the experiments of Eijkman and Grijns.

Grijns compiled the evidence and was able to convince Eijkman of the obvious, that white rice lacked an essential, water-soluble nutrient present in the bran, and that beriberi resulted from a deficiency of that nutrient. Grijns published his findings and conclusion in 1901, unfortunately in an obscure journal and written in Dutch, delaying its dissemination outside of Holland.[6] Even though his impact was delayed, he had proven that beriberi resulted from a nutritional deficiency and introduced a new way to think about disease.

Picking Up the Trail

While the work of Eijkman and Grijns lay fallow, others picked up where Lunin had left off over twenty years earlier. In 1905, a Dutch physician, C. A. Pekelharing gave an address to the Netherlands Medical Society in which he described his experiments which, like those of Lunin, showed that "there is a still unknown substance in milk which, even in very small quantities, is vital to nourishment."[7] He could not purify the substance, so he gave up the line of investigation. Like Grijns, he published his findings in Dutch; and, once again, the language barrier left his work unappreciated outside of Holland.

A turning point occurred at the November 7, 1906, meeting of the Society of Public Analysts. F. Gowland Hopkins, a lecturer in physiologic chemistry at Cambridge University gave a verbose address, most of which concerned the administration of an examination for medicinal chemists.[8] Near the end of the long speech, he shifted topics to make "prognostications" concerning nutrition, which he called "dietetics." Without mentioning Lunin or Pekelharing or citing his source, he stated "no animal can live upon a mixture of pure protein, fat, and carbohydrate, and even when the necessary inorganic material is carefully supplied still the animal cannot flourish." Hopkins hypothesized that rickets and scurvy resulted from the deficiency of unknown dietetic factors, to which he applied the term "minimal qualitative factors."

By the time he gave that speech, Hopkins had begun his own studies of nutrition. He had performed experiments to test the nutritional quality of proteins and introduced an important experimental innovation. He studied young, growing animals and measured their rate of weight gain as an indicator of the effects of dietary manipulations. Compared to using adult animals, this dramatically shortened the experiments. Young rodents showed a decline in growth rate within days, whereas adult animals took weeks to begin losing weight on a vitamin-deficient diet.

Hopkins published the paper for which he was best known in 1912 in the *Journal of Physiology*.[9] The paper gave detailed descriptions of experiments in which he fed young, growing rats various simplified diets and followed their growth curves and general health. He was careful to measure exactly how much the rats ate and to collect urine and feces to document that the food was absorbed from the intestine.

When he fed the rats a mixture of casein (milk protein), starch, cane sugar, lard, and salts, their growth slowed within a few days even though they took in sufficient calories. After two weeks they stopped growing completely, began to lose weight, and died in three to four weeks. If he added a small amount of whole milk—two milliliters, less than 4% of their total food—the rats grew normally.

Hence, Hopkins had confirmed Lunin's and Pekelharing's findings, but by using young, growing rats rather than adult mice. He echoed their conclusions: "Such results make it perfectly clear that synthetic diets may wholly fail to support the growth of rats even when consumption is quantitatively quite adequate, and the figures [the graphs in the paper] show plainly enough that some factor in the diet other than its protein and energy content is indispensable for growth." He changed his term for the unknown factors from "minimal qualitative factors" to "accessory factors." Nomenclature soon became a topic of dispute.

Unlike Lunin and Pekelharing, Hopkins was a member of the Cambridge University faculty and the British scientific establishment. He published in English. Although his work was not truly original, it captured the attention of scientists and helped catalyze the study of nutritional deficiency diseases and the search for the missing micronutrients.

The search became a race and Hopkins had competitors. In the United States, Thomas B. Osborne and Lafayette B. Mendel at Yale University had obtained results quite similar to those of Hopkins. They fed growing rats milk proteins with and without "protein-free milk," which contained milk's inorganic salts and small organic molecules, including vitamins. Their publication preceded that of Hopkins. Hopkins cites their work; but, to establish his own priority, he spends a great deal of time in his paper pointing out methodological weaknesses of the Osborne and Mendel experiments.

Elmer Verner McCollum at the University of Wisconsin also performed experiments on growing rats similar to those of Hopkins.[10] He found that rats required a lipid-soluble factor to attain normal growth and was credited with discovering vitamin A. McCollum later moved to Johns Hopkins University to be the first chair of the Department of Chemical Hygiene. Despite being repeatedly wrong in his pronouncements, he went on to become the most important nutrition researcher in the United States.

Another of Hopkins's rivals was Casimir Funk, a peripatetic Polish-born chemist. As a Jew, he had to leave Poland to obtain a university education in Switzerland. After graduation, accompanied by his wife and daughter, he moved from job to job across Europe, arriving at the Lister Institute in 1910.

An English physician, Dr. Leonard Braddon, a medical officer to the Federated Malay States (the British possessions in Malaysia) was a school friend of Charles Martin. Braddon witnessed firsthand the devastation that beriberi was causing in Indonesia. Based on his own observations, he thought that it was a nutritional disease; and he had become aware of the work of Eijkman and Grijns. He contacted Martin and urged him to undertake work on beriberi at the Lister Institute. Martin took his suggestion and assigned Casimir Funk and Evelyn Ashley Cooper, a new postdoctoral fellow, to the project.

Funk and Cooper used pigeons for their experiments. Pigeons, like chickens, develop leg weakness when fed a diet of white rice. Cooper developed a biological assay to quantify the anti-beriberi substance by testing the ability of measured quantities of various foods to prevent the disease or to rescue pigeons that had become weak eating a diet limited to white rice. He found rice bran, lentils, egg yolk, yeast, and some nuts to be effective.

Funk used the biological assay to attempt to purify the mysterious nutrient and published his preliminary results in 1911.[11] This paper probably spurred Hopkins to publish his own results. Funk never succeeded in purifying the anti-beriberi substance, and the work came to an abrupt halt with the outbreak of World War I when Funk resumed his journey west and moved to the United States.[12] Nevertheless, the biological assay he and Cooper developed laid the foundation for Harriette Chick's entry into nutrition research.

Although he never achieved major discoveries in the laboratory, Funk was one of the first to articulate the existence of vitamins. In a 1911 paper in the *Journal of State Medicine*, a journal long since defunct, he proposed that beriberi, scurvy, rickets, and pellagra were all caused by a deficiency of micronutrients.[13] He made his mark on the history of medicine by coining the term *vitamine*, a portmanteau of the Latin word *vita*, meaning life, and the chemical term *amine*, meaning nitrogen-containing. It turned out that not all vitamines contained nitrogen, but the name caught on. It was later shortened to *vitamin* to appease linguistic purists.[14]

Hopkins took strong issue with the term vitamines and with the implication that Funk had been their discoverer. He championed the term "accessory food factors." For obvious reasons, *vitamin* survived and *accessory food factors* fell into disuse. But Hopkins won the important battle. His 1906 speech, his 1912 paper, and his status as a leader of nutrition research in Great Britain earned him the 1929 Nobel Prize in Physiology or Medicine, which he shared with Eijkman and not with Funk.

Scurvy

The story of scurvy, vitamin C deficiency, is longer and more circuitous than that of beriberi, but it shares key themes. Like beriberi, scurvy was a disease of technological progress. For beriberi, the new technology was the steam-powered milling machines that came into use at the beginning of the nineteenth century. For scurvy, it was improvements in navigation and ship construction in the fifteenth and sixteenth centuries that made long ocean voyages possible and ushered in the Age of Sail.

As European powers exploited that technology to trade with distant countries and acquire far-flung empires, hundreds of thousands of sailors manned ships that often remained at sea for months at a time, cut off from fresh provisions. The typical sailor's diet–hardtack, salted meats, cheese, dried peas and beer—contained no vitamin C. After months at sea their bodies' stores of vitamin C were exhausted and the men were forced to bear the consequences. Scurvy killed far more sailors than battles, storms, and accidents combined.

The eventual proof that scurvy was a nutritional disease, like the discoveries of Eijkman and Grijns, resulted from experiments with a faulty rationale and unexpected findings. Once again, these findings were exploited by investigators intellectually prepared to move beyond the accepted wisdom and take advantage of their fortuitous observations.

The first clear description of scurvy was by the anonymous chronicler of the first voyage of Vasco da Gama, whose ships sailed from Lisbon around the Cape of Good Hope to India and back from 1497 to 1499. After being at sea without fresh fruit or vegetables for almost six months, as they sailed up the east coast of Africa, da Gama's men began to develop a strange disease marked by generalized weakness, pain and swelling in the extremities, swelling of the gums, and eventual death. When the ships anchored in the mouth of the Zambesi River in what is now Mozambique, the surviving men eagerly ate the fruit, especially the oranges, that grew in abundance along the river-bank and rapidly recovered. The story was repeated on their return voyage.

Although in retrospect it is obvious that the oranges were supplying a nutrient that was missing from the shipboard diet, that was not understood at the time. Physicians offered various theories to explain the effect of fruits and vegetables. The lack of understanding of the mechanism of the disease as well as practical consideration meant that navies and merchants failed to improve the diets of their sailors. Scurvy killed a million sailors of Great Britain alone. Civilians deprived of fresh produce in the winter also experienced scurvy, especially during times of famine.

The first landmark in the understanding of scurvy was the publication in 1753 by James Lind of *A Treatise on the Scurvy*. Lind, born and educated in Edinburgh, was a product of the Scottish Enlightenment; he believed that observation and experiment should replace the speculations of ancient Greek sages.

Lind enlisted in the Royal Navy in 1739 and gained extensive experience with scurvy while serving in the Mediterranean. In 1747 he was the ship's surgeon aboard the *Salisbury*, which was patrolling the English Channel. When scurvy began to afflict the crew, he chose twelve common seamen with the disease. He isolated them in the sick bay and subjected them to a land-mark controlled clinical trial. He gave all twelve the standard naval diet and divided them into pairs to receive supplements to that diet. He gave two of the sailors oranges and gave each of the other five pairs supplements such as cider or acidic mouth washes. The two sailors who received the oranges rapidly recovered, but none of the others. He had systematically verified da Gama's observation that oranges cure scurvy.

Despite his belief in the value of experiment, Lind could not completely escape the dominant ideas of his day. To explain the benefit of oranges, he pro-posed a variant of the theory of *miasma*, the belief that diseases were caused by bad air. He blamed scurvy on the humid air on board ships and concocted a complicated theory, proposing that the acid in the oranges unblocked pores and permitted the men to sweat out toxins.

The Admiralty ignored his book. They remained skeptical of the benefit of citrus fruit and were unwilling to accept the expense of supplying fresh fruit to common sailors during long voyages. Lind did not press the issue. He later wrote, "The province has been mine to deliver precepts: the power is in others to comply."[15] For four decades, others did not comply. Lind's report of the first controlled clinical trial in the medical literature, although of great importance in the history of medicine, had virtually no immediate impact on navies or merchant marines. Men continued to die of scurvy.

The next landmark, in contrast, did have an impact. Another Edinburgh trained physician, Gilbert Blane, while serving as chief medical officer of Great Britain's fleet in the West Indies during the Seven Years' War (known in the United States as the French and Indian War), carried out detailed epidemiological studies of the incidence of scurvy on the ships and hospitals under his supervision.[16] In the process, he pioneered the science of clinical epidemiology and his data reinforced Lind's demonstration of the value of citrus fruit. Through persistence and sound science, he persuaded the Admiralty to provide lime juice for its sailors. Principally because of the expense, merchant ships took longer to comply; and Parliament dragged its feet in forcing the issue. Nevertheless, the incidence of scurvy among sailors fell dramatically during the final decades of the eighteenth century and the first decades of the nineteenth.

Another important advance was the description of infantile scurvy by the English pediatrician Thomas Barlow. In his 1883 paper, he described 31 children who had been fed proprietary formulas instead of being breast fed.[17] They suffered developmental delay and pain and swelling in the legs. Prior to Barlow, the disease was thought to have been a form of rickets. However, when Barlow examined fatal cases pathologically he found hemorrhages around the bones and separation of the growing ends of long bones from the shafts, abnormalities that had been described by Lind in young men dying of scurvy. Barlow recognized the disease in infants as scurvy. His paper was a model of clinical and pathological description. Infantile scurvy became known as *Barlow's disease.*

Barlow's pathological observations proved essential in the work that proved that scurvy is a nutritional disease. Late in the nineteenth century, Norwegian sailors returning from Asia began to experience a disease called *ship beriberi,* which in some cases was associated with nerve degeneration but more often resembled scurvy. The Norwegians associated the disease with a change in diet. To improve the palatability of sailors' food on long voyages, they gave them canned meat and vegetables. Without direct evidence, they blamed ship beriberi on bacterial contamination of the tinned foods and the production of an uncharacterized bacterial toxin termed *ptomaine*. They had no way of knowing that the true culprit was heating the foods during the canning process, thereby destroying its vitamin C and thiamin.

In 1907, the Norwegian navy enlisted two researchers, Axel Holst and Theodor Frølich, to investigate the disease. They assumed that the disease was beriberi and began by reproducing Eijkman's experiments using pigeons instead of chickens. They then set out to develop a model of beriberi in mammals. Their good fortune was to select guinea pigs for their experiments, as they, like humans, cannot synthesize their own vitamin C and must obtain it from the diet.

When they fed the guinea pigs the same diet of milled grains that produced beriberi in pigeons, the guinea pigs developed a fatal disease. But when examined pathologically, there was no degeneration of the peripheral nerves. Instead, as Holst and Frølich shrewdly recognized, there were changes in the bones and surrounding tissues similar to those described by Thomas Barlow in infantile scurvy and by Lind in young sailors. Holst and Frølich had created an animal model of scurvy and had proven that its cause was faulty nutrition, the result of a "one-sided diet" in their words.[18] After four centuries, they had proven the cause of scurvy.

Despite many wrong turns, scientists had finally established the causes of beriberi and scurvy; and both could be studied in the laboratory, beriberi in birds and scurvy in guinea pigs. Despite the centuries-long delay, by 1915 the existence of micronutrients, substances present in foods in only minute quantities but essential for health, had become widely accepted, although none had been chemically purified and characterized. The field was poised for rapid progress, not only in scientific understanding but also in contributions to public health. The foundation was laid for Harriette Chick to systematically study vitamins in the laboratory. Responding to the Boss's message from Lemnos, she entered the field at an opportune time.

Notes

1 McCollum, Elmer Verner (1957) *A History of Nutrition.* (Boston: Houghton Mifflin), pp. 75-83.

2 Lunin N (1881) Über die Bedeutung der onorganischen Salze für Ernährung des Thieres. *Hoppe-Seyler Zeit f Physiol Chem* 5: 31-39.

3 Voss HE (1956) Nicolai Lunin 1853-1937. *J Amer Dietetic Assn* 32 (4): 317-320.

4 Carpenter, Kenneth J. (2000) *Beriberi, White Rice, and Vitamin B. A Disease, a Cause and a Cure.* Berkeley: University of California Press.

5 Eijkman C (1929) Antineuritic vitamin and beriberi. Nobel lecture. In: *Nobel Lectures, Physiology or Medicine 1922-1941.* Amsterdam: Elsevier, 1965. [Also available at https://www.nobelprize.org/prizes/medicine/1929/eijkman/lecture/]

6 Grijns G (1901) Over polyneuritis gallinarum. *Geneeskundig Tijdschrift voor Nererlandsch-Indië* 41: 3-110. [Published in English in: Grijns G (1935) *Researches on Vitamins 1900-1911* (Gorinchem: J Noorduyn en Zoon), pp. 1-108.]

7 Quoted by van Leersum EC (1926) The discovery of vitamins. *Science* 64 (1658): 357-358.

8 Hopkins FG (1906) The analyst and the medical man. *The Analyst* 31 (369): 385-404.

9 Hopkins FG (1912) Feeding experiments illustrating the importance of accessory factors in normal dietaries. *J Physiol (Lond)* 44 (5-6): 425-460.

10 McCollum EV, Davis M (1913) The necessity of certain lipins in the diet during growth. *J Biol Chem* 15 (1): 167-175.

11 Funk C (1911) On the chemical nature of the substance which cures polyneuritis in birds induced by a diet of polished rice. *J Physiol* 43 (5): 395-400.

12 Funk C (1911) On the chemical nature of the substance which cures polyneuritis in birds induced by a diet of polished rice. *J Physiol* 43 (5): 395-400.

13 Funk C (1912) The etiology of the deficiency diseases. *J State Med* 20: 341-368 [Reprinted in S. A. Goldblith and M. A. Joslyn (1964) *Milestones in Nutrition.* (Westport CT: Avi Publishing), pp. 145-172.]

14 Drummond JC (1920) The nomenclature of the so-called accessory food factors (vitamins). *Biochem J* 14 (5): 660.

15 Lund, James (1757) *An essay on the Most Effectual Means of preserving the Health of Seamen in the Royal Navy.* (London: A. Millar), p. 107.

16 Blane, Gilbert (1785) *Observations of the Diseases Incident to Seamen.* London: Joseph Cooper.

17 Barlow T (1883) On cases described as "acute rickets" which are probably a combination of scurvy and rickets, the scurvy being an essential, and the rickets a variable element. *Med-Chir Trans* 66: 159-220.

18 Holst A. (1907) Experimental studies relating to "ship beri-beri" and scurvy. I. Introduction. *J Hyg (Lond)* 7 (5): 619-633.

Holst A, Frølich T (1907) Experimental studies relating to ship beri-beri and scurvy: II. On the etiology of scurvy. *J Hyg (Lond)* 7 (5): 634-671.

CHAPTER 6
FEEDING SOLDIERS AND EXPLORERS

Although the new change of direction did not allow Harriette to resume her studies of bacteriology and basic protein chemistry, it relieved her of the routine work preparing sera and gave her the opportunity to do original research. She rapidly assembled a team, by necessity almost all women, to conduct the time-consuming experiments. The exacting work required skilled investigators. Chick's major collaborator was Margaret Hume. Ruth Skelton, E. Marion Delf, and Olive Lodge rounded out the team. All had degrees in science. Marion Delf, an established botanist, interrupted her own career to join the team and contribute to the war effort. The only man on the team, Mr. A. H. Robins, helped feed the animals.

Beriberi

When Charles Martin asked Harriette Chick to take over nutrition research at the Lister Institute, he posed the question of what food the army could include in soldiers' rations to prevent beriberi. Following Funk and Cooper's methods, Chick and her team used pigeons for their experiments. It was tedious and demanding work. The birds had to be housed individually and sometimes fed by hand. The women examined them daily and collected and weighed their uneaten food. Each experiment lasted two to three months.

Harriette Chick presented their findings at a 1917 meeting of the Society of Tropical Medicine and Hygiene.[1] She began by stating the foundation of the work: "Sufficient evidence is now available to permit beriberi and scurvy to be classed among the 'deficiency' diseases due to a defective diet, without further comment." In a footnote, she added: "Rickets and pellagra and some less known diseases of cattle are also generally classed among the diseases due to defective nutrition; investigation in these cases is, however, not nearly so far advanced as in scurvy and beriberi."

She went on to summarize the current understanding of nutrition:

> *For perfect nutrition the human being requires, in addition to an adequate ration of fat, protein, carbohydrate, salts and water, a sufficient supply of accessory food factors or vitamines. These substances have not so far been successfully isolated; little is known of their chemical or physical properties, and, at the present time, their presence can only be detected by biological methods. There are, at least, two distinct classes of these vitamines: (1) the vitamine whose presence in a diet is an essential for the proper nutrition of the nervous system, and whose absence or deficiency will give rise to beriberi: for the sake of brevity this may be called the anti-neuritic or anti-beriberi vitamine; (2) the antiscorbutic vitamine, whose absence or deficiency in a diet will occasion scurvy with its characteristic pathological changes.*

She mentioned the term "accessory food factor" to avoid ruffling the feathers of F. Gowland Hopkins; but she preferred Funk's more succinct "vitamine," which she defined as "any accessory substance necessary for satisfactory metabolism, deficiency of which in a diet will lead to the occurrence of a 'deficiency' disease." She left open the possibility of yet undiscovered vitamines.

To prevent beriberi, she and her coworkers sought a dietary supplement that was inexpensive to prepare, easy to transport, sufficiently compact to carry in a backpack, and resistant to heat and cold. They used the biological assay developed by Cooper and Funk to measure the content of the anti-beriberi vitamin in a wide variety of foods.

The team performed two types of experiments, preventive and curative.

In the preventive experiments, they fed pigeons 40 grams of polished rice daily, a diet which led to the onset of nerve degeneration after 15-25 days. To assess the efficacy of various foods, they added measured amounts of individual foods to the rice diet and judged them to contain the anti-beriberi vitamin if the birds remained healthy for 50-60 days. For the curative experiments, they fed the birds the rice diet until weakness appeared and then tested the ability of individual foods to reverse the disease.

Dr. Chick compared the two methods:

There is no doubt that the most trustworthy results are obtained from the preventive tests. They are, however, very exacting and laborious, the feeding is artificial, and must be continued for about two months, with daily careful supervision. If the inquiry were limited to this type of experiment its scope would be seriously restricted. In considering the values obtained from curative experiments, allowance must be made for a large margin of error, seeing that it is impossible to control the onset of polyneuritis so that the type of symptom and the severity of the condition should always be the same at the time of the administration of the cure.

The team tested a variety of foods, including vegetables, grains and meats. They found the anti-beriberi vitamin to be present to some degree in all foods tested, but in greatest concentration in the seeds of plants and the eggs of animals. Cereals and edible pulses (beans, peas and lentils) were the most effective in curing the birds. In grains, including rice, the highest concentration was in the germ.[2] While it had been assumed that grinding off the bran was responsible for the loss of the anti-beriberi vitamin from milled grains, in reality most of the vitamin was lost with removal of the germ.

Fish was not curative but fish roe was. Cow's milk, cheese and potatoes were poor sources of the vitamin. Important to their future work and to the health of the troops, they found high concentrations in yeast and yeast extract.

They confirmed the finding of Grijns that the anti-beriberi vitamin was relatively stable to heating at 100 degrees Celsius, but not at 120 degrees.[3] This accounted for "ship beriberi," which occurred when the Norwegian navy switched to feeding their sailors canned foods sterilized at 120 C in the canning process.

Yeast powder provided an easily transported source of the anti-beriberi vitamin for the troops, but it tastes terrible. It could be added to soup cubes as a more palatable alternative and is contained in the breakfast spread Marmite, which the British, but only the British, find palatable. After fortified soup cubes were issued to the troops in the Middle East, beriberi disappeared. Harriette Chick and her team had answered Dr. Martin's question and helped preserve the health of the troops.

Scurvy

Scurvy was also a problem for the military, as it afflicted soldiers in the Middle East who were fighting in the desert without access to fresh fruit or vegetables. The Lister Institute team studied that disease using guinea pigs. Even the housekeeper helped out, feeding them after hours.

Harriette presented the scurvy experiments to the Society for Tropical Medicine and Hygiene in the same presentation as the beriberi studies.[4] Following the methods of Holst and Frølich, they fed guinea pigs oats, which led to signs of scurvy in two to three weeks. They also added milk heated to 120 C for one hour to destroy its small content of vitamin C. The heated milk had no effect on the onset of scurvy but maintained the animals in better overall health. Chick does not discuss this observation in detail, but she essentially had repeated the experiments of Lunin and F. Gowland Hopkins demonstrating that milk contains vital nutrients in addition to the anti-beriberi and antiscorbutic factors.

The guinea pig experiments, like those with the pigeons, were laborious and tedious.

The guinea pigs in most cases require a certain amount of hand feeding to gain assurance that the requisite doses of the materials studied are really taken and much care is needed to render the foodstuffs palatable, for many of these studied are far removed from the natural food of this animal, and different treatment is required in each separate case. Further, a good deal of skilled attention is necessary if the general

health and weight of the animal is to be maintained, apart from the
question of scurvy. Under these circumstances the output of work pos-
sible from any one worker is limited..."

Unlike the beriberi experiments in pigeons, all the experiments with
guinea pigs were preventive in design. Dr. Chick's explanation underlines the
attention she and her colleagues devoted to the animals.

There is no particular advantage in the curative type of experiment
where scurvy is concerned. The onset of the disease is gradual and by
the time the symptoms – loss of weight, painful joints and loosening
teeth – are well marked, the lesions are extensive and the animal is in
a weak condition. If, at this stage, a powerful antiscorbutic, such as
orange juice, is given, the cure is extremely slow and it may be many
weeks before the animal may be said to be in perfect health. In fact, it
is doubtful whether the joints ever become perfectly normal, and even
when the cured animals seemed to have reached a thriving condition,
one could frequently detect a slight tenderness of the arm and leg joints
by a careful examination.

The Lister Institute investigators found that the distribution of the
antiscorbutic vitamin was much more restricted than the anti-neuritic substance. Among the foods tested, fresh lemon and lime juice were the best, but
the benefit was rapidly lost when the juices were stored. Harriette surmised
that this explained the reappearance of scurvy among British polar explorers, whereas prior expeditions had escaped the disease. She suggested that
"modern methods of manufacture may have introduced some modification
detrimental to the antiscorbutic principle originally contained." This became
the subject of separate studies.

Cabbage leaves were also an excellent source of the antiscorbutic substance. Onions, carrots, and boiled potatoes proved somewhat less beneficial;
and cow's milk and meat were only weakly antiscorbutic. Unfortunately, yeast
had no value. Unlike the anti-beriberi vitamin, heating to 100 C destroyed the
antiscorbutic factor.[5]

For the troops, Harriette Chick recommended onions and potatoes when available. Dried beans and peas, which she called *pulses*, are not antiscorbutic. However, if soaked in water to germinate for 72 hours, they produce the necessary vitamin. She suggested this as a possibility for the army and included an appendix with detailed instructions for germinating and then cooking peas and beans. Although not practical in the trenches, these methods led to the cure of scurvy in hospitalized Serbian soldiers at the end of World War I.[6]

To complete her presentation, she discussed the relevance of her findings to human experience. She pointed out that white flour, like white rice, lacks the anti-beriberi vitamin. She noted that colonists in Newfoundland suffered from beriberi during the winters when they ate mainly white bread, which they preferred, but not when they were limited to brown bread. The relative nutritional qualities of white and brown bread were to become a major issue during the next world war.

Another example was provided by troops in the Middle East. English soldiers ate white bread and suffered from beriberi. They enjoyed generous rations of fresh meat, which in large amounts prevents scurvy. The Indian soldiers in the same environment ate dhall prepared from beans. As a result, they did not suffer from beriberi. But they refused to eat meat and developed scurvy.

Chick also pointed out that humans deprived of both the anti-beriberi and antiscorbutic factors develop symptoms of scurvy before they develop nerve degeneration. This accounted for the experience of Norwegian sailors fed canned foods, lacking both vitamins. Their "ship beriberi" was predominantly scurvy. Chick also verified that canned foods were a poor source of vitamins.[7]

In the discussion that followed the oral presentation, several members of the audience praised the careful work of the Lister Institute team. Charles Martin, still a lieutenant colonel, remarked on the detailed attention the team devoted to caring for the animals to ensure that the experimental protocols were followed rigorously.

The evidence that Chick and her colleagues amassed eliminated any residual doubt that beriberi and scurvy were diseases of faulty nutrition. No one could find fault with their meticulous attention to experimental method. Even E. V. McCollum came around. As one instance of his propensity to be wrong, he initially refused to believe that rats, which synthesize their own ascorbic acid and do not suffer from scurvy, could differ in their basic nutritional requirements from guinea pigs, which are susceptible to the disease. He had performed experiments in which he found impacted feces in the cecum of scorbutic guinea pigs and concocted a theory of intestinal autointoxication to explain the disease.[8] He recanted when he saw the data from the Lister Institute team.

However, not everyone so easily abandoned their cherished beliefs. After Harriette Chick completed her presentation, two physicians rose to argue that beriberi was an infectious disease. This is just one example of irrefutable evidence failing to change minds.

Lime Juice in the Navy

The Lister Institute team also solved a dilemma posed by the reappearance of scurvy in polar explorers. In the 1850s, a naval expedition spent twenty-seven months in the Arctic and lost only three men after being trapped in the ice for three winters. They took what the Navy called lime juice; but it was, in fact, prepared from Mediterranean lemons. The Navy made no distinction between lemons and limes. This proved to be a fatal error.

In 1875, an expedition led by Captain George Nares set out to the Arctic and had a different experience than the earlier expedition.[9] Two ships, the *Alert* and the *Discovery*, with 121 crewmen sailed up the west coast of Greenland, where they spent the winter trapped in the ice well north of the Arctic Circle. In April 1876, sixteen men under the command of Commander Albert Markham set out on sledges to push as far north as possible. They had taken their daily doses of lime juice on board ship. It was standard naval issue, but now prepared from limes from Monserrat in the West Indies rather than lemons. Furthermore, the juice may have been pumped through copper pipes during bottling. Copper is a potent catalyst for the oxidation of ascorbic acid, destroying its antiscorbutic activity.

Because of the difficulty of thawing liquids in temperatures well below freezing and the belief that the men had left in a well-nourished state, they did not take lime juice on the sledges. Within two weeks, the first signs of scurvy appeared. The men pushed on for another week and turned back. By the time a search party from the ship met them in early June, scurvy had disabled all but four men; and one had died. On returning to the ship, they found that many crew members who had remained with the ships were also suffering from scurvy. By the time the expedition made it back to England, sixty men had scurvy and four had died.

In the late nineteenth and early twentieth century, the race to be first to the poles was the equivalent of the Cold War space race; and it captured the public's attention in a similar fashion. When polar explorers died, the response was like the reaction to the explosion of the space shuttle *Challenger*. Parliament launched a commission of inquiry to find out what had gone wrong.

The commission compared the Nares expedition to the earlier one, which had not suffered major losses from scurvy. The commission blamed the outbreak on the failure to provide lime juice for the sledging parties. They glossed over the occurrence of scurvy among the men who remained on the ships, downing their daily doses.

The report was controversial. Noted scientists of the Royal Geographical Society disputed its conclusions, although for the wrong reasons. Not understanding how easily ascorbic acid is oxidized, they questioned the effectiveness of lime juice and cited other instances in which it had failed to prevent scurvy. One academic physician, C. R Markham, the cousin of Commander Albert Markham, the leader of the sledging expedition, termed the doctrine of dietary antiscorbutics such as lime juice "the last remnant of an obsolete physiology."[10]

They were not the only ones who continued to doubt that scurvy was dietary. Captain Robert Falcon Scott, the most famous British polar explorer, was a prominent dissenter. From 1901 to 1904, he led an expedition to Antarctica. Scurvy was a recurrent problem while his ship lay trapped in ice over two winters. Lime juice was available to the men, but they were not required to take it. A physician member of his crew, Edward A. Wilson, blamed scurvy on ptomaine, the purported toxin produced by bacteria contaminating tinned food.[11] He was surprised that scurvy struck the men even though "every tin of meat [was] examined by sight and smell."

The Lister Institute team had no doubt that scurvy was dietary and tackled the problem by assaying various preparations of lime juice for their antiscorbutic efficacy. They found that fresh lime juice prepared from limes from the West Indies had only one-quarter the antiscorbutic potency of lemon juice prepared from Mediterranean lemons.[12] Samples of the Navy's preserved lime juice lacked any antiscorbutic activity. They also showed that the antiscorbutic value of other foods decreased over time with storage and verified that it was destroyed by heating.

Alice Henderson Smith complemented these laboratory findings with a historical study of the use of antiscorbutics in the Royal Navy.[13] At the end of the eighteenth century, the Navy stopped using citrus juice preserved by heating and began using the juice of lemons or limes either mixed with rum or briefly brought to a boil and bottled under a layer of olive oil. Omitting the prolonged heating of the juice preserved its vitamin C and contributed to the decline in scurvy in the Navy after 1790.

In 1860 the Navy made another change. It had previously obtained lemons from Malta, Spain, and Italy. When warfare disrupted the supply lines in the Mediterranean, the Navy switched to limes from the Caribbean. It also switched to a new preparation of lime juice. In 1867, Lachlan Rose patented a method for preserving lime juice in a concentrated sugar solution rather than alcohol.[14] Rose's Lime Juice later became popular as an ingredient of cocktails, but his first major customer was the Navy. He opened a factory in Leith, Scotland, near the wharves, and expanded his business to London in 1875. Rose obtained his limes from the West Indies.

Alice Henderson Smith's paper, published in 1919, documented that scurvy had all but disappeared among British sailors when the Navy provided them juice of Maltese lemons.[15] However, in the 1860s, when the military switched to juice prepared from West Indian limes, scurvy reappeared among polar explorers and soldiers in the Middle East. The findings of Chick and Hume showed why that switch resulted in scurvy persisting over 400 years after the crew of Vasco da Gama recognized the curative effects of fresh fruit.

Chick's experiments during World War I firmly established beriberi and scurvy as vitamin deficiency diseases and identified the best foods to supply the vitamins that prevent them. These were important results with a great impact on public health. However, it was another vitamin deficiency disease, rickets, which elevated Harriette Chick into the first rank of medical scientists. The study of that disease would take her to war-ravaged Vienna and occupy the next three years of her life.

Notes

1   Chick, H, Hume M. (1917) The distribution among foodstuffs (especially those suitable for the rationing of armies) of the substances required for the prevention of (a) beriberi and (b) scurvy. *Trans Soc Trop Med Hyg* 10 (8): 141-186; *J Royal Army Medical Corps* 29 (2): 121-159.

2   Chick H, Hume M. (1917) The distribution in wheat, rice, and maize grains of the substance, the deficiency of which in a diet causes polyneuritis in birds and beri-beri in man. *Proc Royal Society Lond* 90 (624): 44-60.

3   Chick H, Hume M. (1917) The distribution among foodstuffs (especially those suitable for the rationing of armies) of the substances required for the prevention of (a) beriberi and (b) scurvy. *Trans Soc Trop Med Hyg* 10 (8): 141-186; *J Royal Army Medical Corps* 29 (2): 121-159.

     Chick H, Hume M. (1917) The effect of exposure to temperatures at or above 100° C. upon the substance (vitamin) whose deficiency in a diet causes polyneuritis in birds and beri-beri in man. *Proc Royal Society Lond* 90 (624): 60-68.

4   Chick H, Hume M. (1917) The distribution among foodstuffs (especially those suitable for the rationing of armies) of the substances required for the prevention of (a) beriberi and (b) scurvy. *Trans Soc Trop Med Hyg* 10 (8): 141-186; *J Royal Army Medical Corps* 29 (2): 121-159.

5   Chick H, Hume M. (1917) The distribution among foodstuffs (especially those suitable for the rationing of armies) of the substances required for the prevention of (a) beriberi and (b) scurvy. *Trans Soc Trop Med Hyg* 10 (8): 141-186; *J Royal Army Medical Corps* 29 (2): 121-159.

     Chick H, Hume M. (1917) The effect of exposure to temperatures at or above 100° C. upon the substance (vitamin) whose deficiency in a diet causes polyneuritis in birds and beri-beri in man. *Proc Royal Society Lond* 90 (624): 60-68.

6   Wiltshire, H. W. (1918) A note on the value of germinated beans in the treatment of scurvy, and some points in prophylaxis. *Lancet* 192 (4972): 811-813.

7   Campbell MED, Chick H (1919) I. The antiscorbutic and growth-promoting value of canned vegetables. *Lancet* 194 (5008): 320-322.

8   McCollum EV, Pitz W (1917) The "vitamin" hypothesis and deficiency diseases. *J Biol Chem* 31 (1): 229-253.

9   Henderson Smith A (1919) A historical inquiry into the efficacy of lime juice for the prevention and cure of scurvy. *J Royal Med Corps* 32 (93-116): 188-208.

Wilson LG (1975)The clinical definition of scurvy and the discovery of vitamin C. *J Hist Med Allied Sci* 30 (1): 40-60.

10 Carpenter, Kenneth J. (1986) *The History of Scurvy and Vitamin C* (Cambridge: Cambridge University Press), p. 145.

11 Wilson EA (1905) The medical aspect of the Discovery's voyage to the Antarctic. *Brit Med J* 2 (2323): 77-80.

12 Chick H., Hume EM., Skelton RF, Henderson Smith A (1918) The relative content of antiscorbutic principle in limes and lemons, together with some new facts and some old observations concerning the value of "lime juice" in the prevention of scurvy. *Lancet* 192 (4970): 735-738.

13 Henderson Smith A. (1919) A historical inquiry into the efficacy of lime-juice for the prevention and cure of scurvy. *J Roy Army Med Corps* 32 (93-116): 188-208.

14 Harvie, David I. (2002) *Limeys. The True Story of One Man's War against Ignorance, the Establishment and the Deadly Scurvy* (Stroud, U.K.: Sutton Publishing), pp. 215-224.

15 Henderson Smith A. (1919) A historical inquiry into the efficacy of lime-juice for the prevention and cure of scurvy. *J Roy Army Med Corps* 32 (93-116): 188-208.

CHAPTER 7
MISSION TO VIENNA

Harriette Chick's work in Vienna was the most important of her career. More documentation of these three years has survived than of any other period. In addition to her original scientific papers, she later wrote review articles describing her experience. Importantly, her diaries from these years have been preserved by the Wellcome Library in London. Although the entries are mainly matter-of-fact descriptions of the events of her days, some include her reflections and opinions and complement her published writings. However, they are hand-written, some entries are sloppy—likely made at the end of the day—and, even at best, her handwriting can be difficult to decipher.

Her trip to Vienna was an initiative of the Medical Research Council. In 1913 the British government formed the Medical Research Committee, later renamed the Medical Research Council (MRC), to advance medical science. In 1918, Walter Morley Fletcher, the Secretary of the MRC, recognizing the importance of the "new science of nutrition," asked five nutrition experts to compile a summary of the recent discoveries about vitamins.[1]

The group first met on May 6, 1918. The Cambridge professor F. Gowland Hopkins chaired the group, so it was named the Accessory Food Factors Committee, using his terminology rather than *vitamine*, the word coined by his rival Casimer Funk. Harriette Chick served as Secretary. In 1919, the Committee issued its *Report on the present state of Knowledge concerning*

Accessory Food Factors (Vitamines).[2] The review was widely read by British physicians and the Committee published two updates in 1924 and 1932.[3]

In addition to summarizing what was already known, the Accessory Food Factors Committee wanted to promote new research. They saw an opportunity in the descriptions filtering into England of widespread famine in Eastern Europe. Harriette Chick had established her credentials as the leading British nutrition scientist and the Committee asked her to go to Vienna to "ascertain to what extent the recent discoveries of vitamin deficiencies in experimental animals were applicable to the human subject."[4]

Accepting the assignment was not an easy decision. Austria was decimated by the war. In addition to concerns about her personal safety, Harriette had to ascertain whether scientific research was feasible in such an environment. She talked to travelers returning from Eastern Europe who verified the severity of the food shortages. She learned that the former chair of pediatrics at Johns Hopkins University, Prof. Clemens von Pirquet, was the director of the Vienna University Kinderklinik, a pediatric inpatient ward of the University of Vienna. He could be a key resource, but he did not believe that vitamins were essential nutrients and "has a very unconventional theory of nutrition."[5]

Charles Martin, Harriette's most important adviser, argued against her going. Aside from concerns about her safety and the feasibility of the project, he would be deprived of her help while she was away and her laboratory would lie fallow. But, gaining the financial backing of the MRC and the Lister Institute, she decided to take the risk. "I took the Boss for a walk in Battersea Park and had my say."[6] But he remained "difficult and unsympathetic."[7]

An experienced clinician, Dr. Elsie Jean Dalyell, an Australian physician working at the Lister Institute on a fellowship, accompanied Harriette. Dr. Dalyell was used to working under difficult conditions, having spent the war serving in the Royal Army Medical Corps in Greece, Malta, and Turkey. The two women set out on September 7, 1919, planning to spend the winter in Vienna to assess the situation. Another colleague, Margaret Hume, joined them in February.

Taking the train across Europe, Harriette Chick stopped in Paris. "We spent a charming day under the trees" in the Bois de Boulogne. "After dinner I was taken out to see the nightlife of Paris, but there wasn't any in our respectable quarter, and I was very tired."[8] She continued on, peeved that the Swiss would only grant her a transit visa and not allow her to get off the train. She arrived in Vienna on September 12.

The Vienna that the women encountered was a different city than Harriette had experienced in 1901 while working with Prof. von Gruber. Vienna at the turn of the century was the political capital of a thriving Austro-Hungarian Empire and a cultural capital of Europe, a modern, prosperous, vibrant city of music, poetry, cafés, and coffee shops. The city shared the new century's optimism. Increasing prosperity raised hopes of ending poverty. Science was broadening its reach; Sigmund Freud had made even the deepest recesses of the human mind a subject of study. Barriers—between social classes, between the sexes and between countries—were breaking down. European powers had not gone to war with each other for a generation and one could travel freely throughout the continent without a passport. Everyone expected the era of peace and progress to continue indefinitely.

Instead, the Great War fractured and devastated Europe. The Hapsburg Empire collapsed. A shaky Austrian republic replaced the monarchy and struggled to maintain order. Vienna had not been a battleground and survived physically intact but economically ruined. It was a brave act for unaccompanied women to spend the winter in the city. They had to bring warm clothes, which were unavailable in Vienna; and fuel to heat buildings was all but unobtainable. On the train, they had to keep an eye on their luggage since theft was rife. To arrange food and lodging they were depending on Harriette Chick's contacts, their status as special guests, and the financial support of the MRC and the Lister Institute.

Austria had suffered food shortages throughout the war. After the war, the situation became even more desperate, especially in cities. Hungary, which had fed its neighbor while the Empire was intact, grew hostile and held onto its produce to feed its own population. The war had decimated agriculture within Austria. The government rationed food and little was for sale in stores. Farmers hoarded their meager crops to sell on the black market, where only the rich could afford to shop. And even they were suffering, as rampant inflation eroded their fortunes and barter replaced the increasingly worthless currency.

In the face of all the privations, the travelers from England had the advantage of bringing British pounds sterling. Although the Viennese were starving, foreigners came to the city to take advantage of favorable exchange rates. Surrounded by destitution, the fashionable shops, cafés, restaurants, and theaters were doing good business. Harriette Chick stayed at the Astoria Hotel, dined out, and attended orchestra concerts and the opera. For foreigners, especially for music lovers, Vienna still had its pleasures.

Post-War Famine

Although she could enjoy the city's attractions, Harriette Chick found the situation for most Viennese even worse than rumored. Upon arriving in the city, she observed:

> *The general impression made by the population as seen in the streets of Vienna in the autumn of 1919, twelve months after the armistice, was great depression matched by slow fatigued movements, and pallid yellow faces. Rarely did one meet a child or grown person with a healthy or rosy complexion.*[9]

British and American relief agencies and the Society of Friends were just beginning to import food from the United States and had not yet made a major impact. Some fresh fruits and vegetables were available in markets, but at prices so high that the poor could not buy them. Children, needing enough food to nourish growing bodies, were especially vulnerable. A survey found that 75% of children in all of Austria and 96% in Vienna were undernourished.[10]

Milk was scarce, so infants suffered disproportionately. Most dairy cattle had been slaughtered for food or shipped to surrounding countries under the punitive terms of the peace treaty. The government banned the sale of milk to the public, reserving the meagre supply for infants and institutionalized children. To compound the problem, the system of transportation was in disarray and milk had to be heated to keep it from spoiling during the three or four days required to bring it from the farm to the city, reducing its content of vitamins.

The result was that most children suffered from multiple vitamin

deficiencies. The shortage of fresh fruit and vegetables during the winter produced vitamin C deficiency and made infantile scurvy common in the spring.
After weaning and being deprived of cows' milk, infants became deficient in
the fat-soluble vitamins A and D. Vitamin A deficiency caused night blindness and corneal ulcerations, and vitamin D deficiency caused rickets.

Virtually all the children had rickets, which was, like scurvy, especially
severe in the spring. Many children suffered from both diseases, which
impacted their growing bones. Scurvy made movement painful and rickets
stunted growth and deformed limbs. The children suffered developmental
delay. Harriette Chick saw the consequences: "It was not unusual to find children of normal weight at birth, who in their first two years had suffered more
than one attack of scurvy, and at this age were about half the normal weight,
could neither sit nor stand without support, made no attempt at speech and
gave little sign of awakened intelligence."[11]

Austrian physicians, deprived of international scientific journals and
communication during the war, knew nothing of vitamins. They thought that
scurvy and rickets were similar to tuberculosis: a chronic infection worsened
by malnutrition and crowded, unsanitary living conditions. Not understanding the need for vitamins, they concentrated on providing children a carbohydrate-rich diet by giving them extra sugar, thinking that sufficient calories
in any form would be adequate for normal growth and development. Before
the invention of antibiotics, they could offer no treatment for the chronic
infections they believed caused rickets and scurvy.

Rickets, the English Disease

Harriette Chick was familiar with the clinical and pathological features of
infantile scurvy from the classic descriptions of the London physician Thomas
Barlow.[12] (The Viennese assumed that Barlow was Russian and called the disease Barloff's disease. Harriette, presumably with tongue in cheek, followed
the local custom while in Vienna.) Both infantile scurvy and rickets affect the
bones, but scurvy causes pains in the joints and legs, whereas rickets is pain-
less. Moreover, rickets has a characteristic appearance on X-rays of the joints.

Harriette Chick had made herself the world's leading authority on
scurvy, studying the disease in guinea pigs and monkeys. She knew it to be a

deficiency of a water-soluble micronutrient. Although she did not know what that nutrient was, she knew what foods supplied it and how to prevent and cure the disease. She did not need to come to Vienna to study scurvy.

But she had a less complete understanding of rickets, and post-war Vienna presented her an unmatched opportunity to study the disease since it afflicted most of the infants in the city. Rickets was a disease of the Industrial Revolution. It was called *the English disease* because it was first described by the seventeenth century English physicians Daniel Whistler and Francis Glisson when it became common in London. By the nineteenth century, it had become widespread among children in industrial cities of Britain, Europe and North America. It had a distinctive epidemiology, being more common in the north of Europe than the south, more common in urban than rural areas, and most severe in the spring.

Rickets typically begins during the first year of life and interferes with the development of growing bones, which become soft and easily deformed. A child with advanced rickets has a characteristic appearance. Growth is stunted. The skull is thin and the fontanelles, the soft spots in an infant's skull, fail to close. The forehead becomes prominent (*frontal bossing*) and the joints enlarge. Especially striking are the joints between the ribs and the sternum, which form a string of protuberances on the chest termed a *rachitic rosary*.

When the child is old enough to bear weight, the leg bones bend and the child becomes either knock-kneed or bandy-legged. The spine may become curved. When the disease is severe, the child is lethargic and misses intellectual milestones. The bony deformities persist throughout life. In northern cities men and women with short stature and crooked legs were common.

Rickets is now known to result from a deficiency of vitamin D, which is required for the absorption of calcium from the intestine and for bones to calcify properly. Bones grow by first adding cartilage. The cartilage then calcifies, forming hard bone, a process that requires calcium, phosphorus, and vitamin D. Rachitic bones add cartilage, but cannot convert the cartilage into mineralized bone, leaving the bones weak and with a characteristic appearance on X-ray.

One can obtain vitamin D from the diet; but prior to the supplementation of cows' milk with the vitamin, the main source was the skin. Ultraviolet light from sunlight converts a form of cholesterol into active vitamin D. Children in northern cities, kept indoors during cold winters and shaded from the summer sun by industrial air pollution, were the most vulnerable to the disease. In England, the burning of coal tripled between 1850 and the beginning of World War I and smoke billowed from the chimneys of factories and private homes.[13] A black cloud covered much of the north of England, obscuring the sun year-round. London and Manchester were especially dark. In the British Isles, rickets was primarily a disease of industrial cities.[14] The same pattern prevailed in Europe and North America.

Before the role of ultraviolet light was understood, there were three prominent theories of rickets. Some, including physicians in Vienna, thought it was a chronic infection like tuberculosis. This fit with the vogue of invoking the germ theory to explain all diseases and the belief that malnutrition weakened the immune system and made people vulnerable to infections.

Physicians and scientists in Glasgow aggressively championed their own theory, that the disease was a consequence of confinement and lack of exercise. They had found that puppies fed only oatmeal and milk and kept indoors developed rickets; but if allowed to run freely outdoors, they recovered. Unaware of the effects of sunlight, the Glaswegians thought exercise to be the cure and pugnaciously refuted the nutritional theory favored by the Londoners at the Lister Institute.

Immersed in vitamin research, Harriette Chick and her colleagues were impressed by reports of dietary cures of rickets in animals, especially the work of Edward Mellanby.[15] A former student of F. Gowland Hopkins, Mellanby was a nutrition researcher at Kings College for Women in London and one of the founding members of the Accessory Food Factors Committee. Beginning in 1916, he tested a variety of diets in puppies. When he fed them milk and oatmeal or milk and bread and kept them indoors, they developed rickets. If he added animal fat, butter or cod liver oil to their diet, they remained healthy. Linseed oil was of no benefit, nor was indoor exercise.[16]

Mellanby was not the first to treat rickets with cod liver oil. He was unaware of the writings of the prominent French physician, Armand Trousseau, who had reported the benefit of cod liver oil for rickets in 1861, but whose account made no impact on medical practice.[17] However, Mellanby did know of the experience of John Bland-Sutton, a surgeon with an interest in comparative anatomy who performed necropsies at the London Zoo. Bland-Sutton gave a presentation to the Zoological Society in 1889 in which he reported that lion cubs brought to the zoo and kept indoors frequently died with rickets, but that it could be prevented by feeding them bone meal and cod liver oil.[18]

Cod liver oil and fish oil were also folk remedies used for a variety of diseases, especially rheumatism, and were popular in Scandinavia and the north of Scotland. These uses received occasional mention in the medical literature but were generally dismissed as superstition.[19]

In 1916, while Mellanby was conducting his studies in dogs, Alfred Hess, a remarkable man in his own right, and his colleague Lester Unger were testing the ability of cod liver oil to prevent rickets in African-American children in New York City. Dark skinned children living in northern cities were especially liable to suffer rickets, as skin pigment blocks ultraviolet rays. In some neighborhoods of New York, over 90 percent of African-American babies suffered rickets.

In their paper of 1917, Hess and Unger did not cite any specific previous work but merely stated, "For many years cod liver oil has been regarded as the sovereign remedy for rickets."[20] To test this belief, they provided cod liver oil to 80 mothers to give to their babies. Many mothers were unable to comply and were either dropped from the study or their babies were continued to be followed to serve as a control group. Of the 49 children who received cod liver oil for four to six months, four-fifths improved compared to none of 16 in the control group. Although as a clinical trial the study suffered from many flaws, the results supported the benefit of cod liver oil.

Hellen M. M. Mackay, a physician who worked with Harriette Chick at the Lister Institute, attempted to carry out similar studies of the dietary treatment of rickets in outpatients in two hospitals in London. However, she despaired of carrying out rigorous studies of dietary deficiencies in outpatients:

My results go to prove the impossibility of obtaining data of sufficient accuracy from out-patient work to give any conclusive results. There was a very wide margin of error in the histories given me; irregular attendances, intercurrent illnesses, and radical changes by the mother in the food (which, perhaps, in spite of careful questioning, I only discovered weeks later), also invalidated many of my records. These sources of error point to the absolute necessity that an investigation in clinical work undertaken with a view to elucidating the cause of a supposed dietetic disorder should be institutional.[21]

Despite her reservations, her observations were consistent with the view that rickets occurred in infants given diets high in carbohydrates and low in fat and that the disease was especially common in bottle-fed infants. A few of her patients improved when the mothers were given cod liver oil to administer to their children. But then it was summer, and Dr. Mackay did not know for sure if the improvement was due to diet or was just the usual seasonal variation in the severity of the disease. She leaned on the side of cod liver oil.

None of the investigators knew what ingredient in cod liver oil and other fats was responsible for its benefit. Mellanby thought it was a factor called *fat-soluble A*. In a landmark 1913 paper, E. V. McCollum and Marguerite Davis at the University of Wisconsin reported that an ingredient in butterfat is required for young rats to grow normally. They called the unknown ingredient fat-soluble A.[22] As McCollum was to discover in 1922, it was a mixture of two vitamins, now called vitamin A and vitamin D, but initially it was assumed to be a single compound.[23]

None of this biochemistry was understood in 1919 when Drs. Chick and Dalyell arrived in Vienna. But they came armed with their new knowledge of nutrition and eager to test their theories in human subjects.

Getting Down to Work

Harriette's first weeks in Vienna were spent carrying out reconnaissance, touring clinics to find patients for clinical trials and relief agencies to get the foods to feed to those patients to test her theories.

Soon after arriving, she visited Professor von Pirquet in his Kinderklinik, a pediatric hospital and research facility supported by the University of Vienna. It was housed in a modern building. The inpatient facilities were spacious, clean and brightly lit; and, importantly for the study of a bone disease like rickets, the X-ray facilities were up to date. The hospital was well staffed: in addition to the director, twelve senior and seven junior medical staff, 120 nurses and 70 domestic staff cared for 100 children. And Dr. von Pirquet was welcoming. Although he was skeptical of Chick's ideas about vitamins, he was eager to promote nutrition research. He offered to make his staff and facilities available for her work and even put his personal car and driver at her disposal. His support proved essential to her success.

The Landes Zentral Kinderheim, directed by Dr. Gustav Riether, presented a contrast to the Kinderklinik. Instead of a well-supported university research facility, it was a public "foundling hospital" housing 400-500 infants, many with their mothers. Newborns were admitted to the pediatric ward directly from the obstetrics service during their first weeks of life; orphans were admitted as infants.

The wards were modern and spacious; but there were few nurses. They supervised the wards and charted the children's growth, development, and diet but could not provide direct care. Instead, the mothers who lived on the wards cared for the children, their own as well as the orphans. No coal was available, so there was no central heating and everybody crowded into interior rooms to keep warm. American relief agencies supplied much of the food, but problems with transportation made the milk supply inconsistent. This was not a suitable environment for controlled clinical trials but it allowed Dr. Dalyell to observe untreated rickets and clarify some of its clinical and radiographic features.[24]

Harriette visited the American Child Feeding Center, which provided food for a thousand children. Each child received 660 calories daily, mainly from beans, flour, cocoa and condensed milk. The food was prepared in a well-equipped kitchen, but the vegetables were overcooked, destroying their vitamins. Harriette also visited several smaller clinics and relief agencies, but she made no further mention of them.

Later, in the spring, Harriette made brief trips to Warsaw and Budapest. In Warsaw, although over half of the children had rickets, food was more available than in Vienna.

At the beginning of May two of us (H. C. and E. J. D.) travelled to Warsaw to inquire into the food situation in Poland and possible existence of deficiency diseases. We found the food situation incomparably better than in Austria, and although prices were high, the shortage of milk and butter appeared to be less and these articles of food could be bought openly in the shops. From casual observation in the streets of Warsaw the ordinary people appeared to be better nourished than in Vienna, they had much better complexions and healthy plump children were everywhere to be seen.[25]

A Productive Winter

After getting the lay of the land, it was clear to Drs. Chick and Dalyell that the Kinderklinik offered the best site for their studies. In December, they took advantage of Dr. von Pirquet's hospitality and got to work. They collected enough food to supplement the diets of a few children. Harriette noted in her diary: "Two children who remain stationary in weight on their diet of milk and sugar are to have a trial of tomato juice and cod liver oil. This is the thin end of the wedge."[26]

The visitors accomplished two dramatic cures. They first cured a child of infantile scurvy with lemon juice. No oranges were to be had and the infant could not tolerate acidic lemon juice. To make it palatable, the women had to laboriously concentrate the juice in a vacuum and neutralize its acidity with chalk.

They then cured a corneal ulcer in a child by supplementing the diet with butterfat, which they were able to obtain from the Society of Friends. Corneal ulceration (*keratomalacia*) is a sign of vitamin A deficiency. Vitamin A occurs in two forms: one fat-soluble and contained in milk, eggs and meat, the other water-soluble and contained in vegetables such as carrots, sweet potatoes and green, leafy vegetables. Since these all were in short supply, vitamin A deficiency was a common cause of blindness in post-war Europe.

The Londoners, with their novel ideas about nutrition, were first received with "polite incredulity" by Viennese doctors, but these initial successes gave them credibility.[27] The influential cardiologist Karel Frederic Wenckebach, professor at the University of Vienna and director of its medical clinic, was receptive to their ideas. Born and educated in Holland, he had read Eijkman's work on beriberi, originally published in a Dutch journal. He invited the women to his house to give an informal talk to update some of his colleagues on the new discoveries about vitamins.

Harriette Chick gave the talk in German, as she had become fluent during her studies in Munich and Vienna. The talk went well and prompted Wenckebach to arrange a formal presentation to the entire medical society in the lecture hall at his clinic. That talk was well attended and earned the Londoners the support of the local doctors.

Harriette was encouraged by her reception. Rather than being deterred by the risks of working in a war-scarred city, she recognized a unique opportunity to test the new ideas about nutrition. Ever the rational scientist, she saw that the ravages of war would allow her to verify in humans the results from animal studies.

Conditions of acute food shortage have the great advantage for experimental investigation that they inexorably provide what science calls 'negative controls,' or a series of individuals left untreated for purposes of comparison. For ethical reasons such a group of human subjects cannot be created artificially to serve a scientific experiment, but can be utilized if they occur naturally.[28]

The Kinderklinik, was an excellent environment for her studies, as it was rigidly organized and the staff devoted a great deal of attention to nutrition. Most of the infants were breastfed for a few months after birth and then switched to a diet of diluted cow's milk with added sugar. The milk was generally days old and had been heated at least once to keep it from spoiling. As the children matured, first cereal and then overcooked vegetables were added to their diet.

To minimize wasting milk in the face of the severe shortage, Prof. von Pirquet had developed his NEM system to ensure that the children received sufficient calories. The standard food value was the "Nem," the average caloric value of one milliliter of human or cow's milk. In the clinic's kitchen, the caloric value of the milk was measured daily and adjusted by adding cane sugar. The Nem requirement of each child was calculated based on age, size, and activity level. An elaborate record-keeping system charted each child's daily food intake, weight, physical activity, and clinical condition.

Despite receiving the required calories based on the NEM system, the diet was deficient in vitamin C and the fat-soluble vitamins A and D. Consequently, almost all the children in the hospital had rickets and had suffered attacks of scurvy. They were far below normal in length and weight and, more distressingly, were listless and lagging in their motor and intellectual development. However, the NEM system and the rigid organization of the clinic ensured that each child received a standard diet with adequate calories and that detailed records of each child's weight, height and diet were maintained. It was an ideal environment for nutrition research, especially to study the effects of supplementing the vitamin-deficient diet with other foods. Because there was not enough food available to supplement the diets of all the children, the Kinderklinik provided an abundance of negative controls.

Drs. Chick and Dalyell worked at the Kinderklinik from December 1919 until June 1920. They spent much of their time and energy procuring vitamin-rich foods from relief agencies. They managed to get enough to supplement the diet of nine children twelve to thirty-one months of age.[29] To prevent scurvy, they obtained a truckload of swede turnips (rutabaga). Their prior work at the Lister Institute had shown swede turnips to be a good source of vitamin C and they fed the children turnip juice, supplemented with neutralized lemon juice when available.[30] To provide fat-soluble vitamins, they gave the children cod liver oil and butter.

Within weeks, all nine children on the enriched diets gained weight and started to catch up in their growth. Their fontanelles closed. The most striking improvements were in motor and intellectual function. Four children could not sit unsupported when the study began but could do so within three months of improved nutrition.

One girl by twenty-eight months of age had shown dramatic improvement. She was discovered to have a twin brother on another ward who had not had the benefit of an enriched diet. A photograph of the chubby and bright-eyed little girl sitting next to her short, skinny twin requiring support by the hands of an adult provided a dramatic illustration for the paper.

An Ill-fated Attempt at Charity

Harriette was touched by the plight of the Viennese children and, with a strong Victorian sense of duty, she initially saw her role as wider than merely conducting research. "I have been paying visits and carrying out a certain amount of unofficial relief work – as I have a general, though perhaps superficial knowledge of conditions in the city."[31] She became involved with a short-lived effort called the Famine Area Children's Hospitality Committee. The organization's mission was to bring children from Eastern Europe to England to live with volunteer host families for up to a year, attending school, learning English, and experiencing the English way of life.

Harriette took on the task of interviewing mothers to identify children for the program. She exchanged letters with Mr. and Mrs. Ensor, who represented the organization back in England, discussing which children were suitable for the program. Social class was the primary issue, and they agreed that middle-class children were the best candidates. Harriette wrote on May 14, 1920: "Of the children we saw yesterday less than 5% were of any other than the industrial class, and at the moment this is just the class that is relatively best off. Though wage and price do not keep pace, they are not as tragically out of proportion as price and any form of fixed income."[32] Furthermore, "In all these troubles of life and daily provision of food etc. people of the middle class are still most keen to provide good educational advantages for their children and they welcome the opportunity of sending their children for 6 months or a year to England."

On May 28 she wrote in her diary of a conversation with a doctor whose name is illegible. She described him as "a broad minded and intelligent man." "He said it will not be wise to state publicly that the English hospitality is offered to middle-class children only." Despite her concern for the children, Harriette could not escape the classicism of her time and culture.

However, only one train filled with children was dispatched to England. When Harriette learned that additional trains were canceled, she wrote to the Ensors and did not mince words: "We feel that one has in a way broken faith with these people." She wrote no more about her unofficial relief efforts, which she presumably abandoned in frustration.

Looking to the Future

Harriette Chick, assisted by Elsie Dalyell and Margaret Hume, had gotten off to a good start during her nine months in Vienna. She had established excellent relations with the Viennese medical community and had managed to get enough supplemental nutrients to perform uncontrolled clinical studies and help a few children in the process. The food situation was slowly improving and she was optimistic that relief agencies could provide sufficient food for additional studies.

Her observations, although not based on rigorous controlled trials, reinforced the importance of vitamins in the growth and development of infants. But in 1920, before the vitamins had been purified and chemically identified, some physicians still doubted their importance. Harriette needed more rigorous evidence to convince the skeptics. She and her colleagues had shown that, despite the deprivations of the war, they could do good clinical science with the support of von Pirquet and his staff. The women were eager to continue the work and returned to London to prepare for more studies.

Notes

1   Chick H, Hume EM (1956) The work of the Accessory Food Factors Committee. *Brit Med Bull* 12 (1): 5-8.

2   Medical Research Committee (1919) *Report on the present state of Knowledge concerning Accessory Food Factors (Vitamines)*. London, His Majesty's Stationery Office.

3   Medical Research Council (1924) *Report on the Present State of Knowledge of Accessory Food Factors (Vitamins)*. London: His Majesty's Stationery Office.

    Medical Research Council (1932) *Vitamins: A Survey of Present Knowledge*. London: His Majesty's Stationery Office.

4   Chick H (1945) Nutritional researches in Vienna after the First World War. *Proc Nutrition Soc* 3 (1): 59-67.

5   Chick, H., personal diary, Wednesday, August 13, 1919. Wellcome Library, London.

6   Chick H, personal diary, Thursday, May 22, 1919, and Saturday August 30, 1919. Wellcome Library, London.

7   Chick H, personal diary, Saturday, August 30, 1919. Wellcome Library, London.

8   Chick H, personal diary, Tuesday, September 9, 1919. Wellcome Library, London.

9   Chick H (1945) Nutritional researches in Vienna after the First World War. *Proc Nutrition Soc* 3 (1): 59-67.

10   Chick H. (1945) Nutritional researches in Vienna after the First World War. *Proc Nutrition Soc* 3 (1): 59-67.

11   Chick H (1945) Nutritional researches in Vienna after the First World War. *Proc Nutrition Soc* 3 (1): 59-67.

12   Barlow T. On cases described as "acute rickets" which are probably a combination of scurvy and rickets, the scurvy being an essential, and the rickets a variable element. *Med Chir Trans* 66 (1883): 159-220.

13   Reed P (2021) Alfred Fletcher's campaign for black smoke abatement, 1864–96: Anticipating the 1956 Clean Air Act. *Ine J Hist Engin Tech* DOI: 10.1080/17581206.2021.1985388. Available at: https://doi.org/10.1080/17581206.2021.1985388.

14   Owen I (1889) Geographical distribution of rickets, acute and subacute rheumatism, chorea, cancer, and urinary calculus in the British islands. *Br Med J* 1: 113-116.

15   Mellanby E (1918) The part played by an "accessory factor" in the production of experimental rickets. *Proc Physiol Soc* (January 26, 1918) xi-xii.

     Mellanby E (1918) A further demonstration of the part played by accessory food factors in the ætiology of rickets. *Proc Physiol Soc* (December 14, 1918) liii-liv.

16   Mellanby, Edward (1921) *Experimental Rickets.* Medical Research Council Special Report No. 61. London: H. M. Stationery Office.

17   Dunn PM (1999) Professor Armand Trousseau (1801-67) and the treatment of rickets. *Arch Dis Child Fetal Neonatal Ed* 80: F155-F157.

18   Bland-Sutton J (1889) *J Comp Med Surg* 10: 1.

19   Guy RA (1923) The history of cod liver oil as a remedy. *Am J Dis Child* 26 (2): 112-116.

20   Hess AF, Unger LJ (1917) Prophylactic therapy for rickets in a negro community. *J Amer Med Assn* 69 (19): 1583-1586.

21   Mackay HMM (1920) Observation on cases of rickets in an out-patient department. *Br Med J* 2 (3129): 929-932.

22   McCollum EV, Davis M (1913) The necessity of certain lipins in the diet during growth. *J Biol Chem* 15 (1): 167-175.

23   McCollum EV, Simmonds N, Becker JE, Shipley PG (1922) Studies on experimental rickets. XXI. An experimental demonstration of the existence of a vitamin which promotes calcium deposition. *J Biol Chem* 53 (2): 293-312.

24   Medical Research Council (1923) *Studies of Rickets in Vienna 1919-22.* (London: H. M. Stationary Office), pp. 130-138.

25   Chick H, Dalyell EJ, Hume EM (1920) Third report of investigation upon deficiency

diseases in Vienna. Report to the Accessory Food Factors Committee. National Archives of Great Britain.

26   Chick H, personal diary, Tuesday, October 14, 1919.

27   Chick H (1976). Study of rickets in Vienna 1919-1922. *Med Hist* 20: 41-51.

28   Chick, Harriette; Hume, Margaret; and Macfarlane, Marjorie (1971) *War on Disease. A History of the Lister Institute.* (London: Andre Deutsch), p. 155.

29   Chick H, Dalyell EJ (1921). Observations on the influence of foods rich in accessory factors in stimulating development in backward children. *Br Med J* 2 (3182): 1061-1066.

30   Chick H, Rhodes M (1918) An investigation of the antiscorbutic value of the raw juices of root vegetables with a view to their adoption as an adjunct to the dietary of infants. *Lancet* 192 (4971): 774-775.

31   Letter to Mr. and Mrs. Ensor dated 14 May 1920. Wellcome Library, London.

32   Letter to Mr. and Mrs. Ensor dated 14 May 1920. Wellcome Library, London.

CHAPTER 8

TWO MORE YEARS IN VIENNA

The Londoners came home in June of 1920 and wrote up their preliminary observations for publication in the *British Medical Journal*.[1] Their work had impressed the Viennese doctors and their ideas had started to seem less radical. Dr. von Pirquet wrote to invite them back to Vienna to conduct formal clinical trials of their treatment for rickets. He remained skeptical of their ideas about nutrition, still clinging to the belief that rickets was infectious; but he respected the women's hard work and did not think cod liver oil would harm his patients.

Harriette spent much of her summer securing financial backing. She managed to obtain sufficient support from the MRC, the Lister Institute, and the Red Cross to support two more years of work. In the Fall of 1920, she took an expanded team back to Vienna. To help with large clinical trials, Margaret Hume, Helen M. M. Mackay, and Hannah Henderson Smith joined her. All had worked in Harriette's laboratory. Helen Mackay, an experienced physician, along with Elsie Dalyell, provided clinical expertise.

Rigorous Science

Pirquet continued to be a generous host. He made a ward of twenty beds in the Kinderklinik available for the rickets experiments. A forty-bed pavilion added to the Meidling Hospital in a southern suburb of Vienna, also under the direction and rigid dietary control of Dr. von Pirquet, enabled the study

of up to sixty infants at one time. Harriette noted that the Kinderklinik was
an ideal facility for the clinical trials:

> It is clear that effective clinical investigation dealing with the relation
> of diet to incidence of rickets can only be carried out under conditions
> in which strict control of diets, both quantitative and qualitative, can
> be exercised. The University Kinderklinik, under the direction of Prof.
> Pirquet, provided special facilities for quantitative work. For some
> years, the research work carried on in this institution has been largely
> devoted to the subject of nutrition in childhood, and in the development
> of Prof. Pirquet's NEM system, methods of allotting, controlling, and
> recording diets have been especially elaborated. The staff has received a
> degree of training and experience in the technical details of nutritional
> work, which is probably without parallel elsewhere.[2]

Helen Mackay, frustrated in her attempts to carry out studies of cod liver
oil in an outpatient clinic, thought the rigorous study of dietary deficiencies
had to be institutional; here was the perfect institution.[3]

The first clinical trial began in November 1920 and continued through
the following summer. It was straightforward in design but produced an
unexpected result. The study compared the ability of two diets to prevent
rickets, one high in carbohydrates and the other high in fat, including cod
liver oil. All the infants in the trial were housed under similar conditions and
received otherwise identical care. When admitted to the study, they ranged in
age from one week to five months; none had signs of rickets.

One group, the controls (the "Pirquet babies"), received Diet I, the standard hospital diet of cows' milk and sugar up to the age of five months, when
cereal and later fresh fruits and vegetables were added. The experimental
group (the "English babies") received Diet II with the same caloric value as
Diet I but with less carbohydrate and more fat, including up to eight grams
per day of cod liver oil. Both groups received the juice of lemons, tomatoes,
or swede turnips to prevent scurvy. To complicate matters, beginning in the
spring, all the children were taken outside into the sunshine when the weather

permitted. Harriette Chick wrote in retrospect, "It was not then known that such a procedure could have any significance."[4]

Taking advantage of the Kinderklinik's excellent X-ray equipment, the investigators based the diagnosis of rickets on radiologic examination of the legs, a more objective measure than clinical examination. They followed 51 children for 5 to 15 months. The first results were unsurprising. Fourteen of the 24 Pirquet babies receiving Diet I developed rickets over the winter, but none of the English babies on Diet II containing cod liver oil. Younger infants on Diet I appeared more susceptible than the older ones. This was what the Lister Institute workers expected, fitting with their belief that rickets was caused by a nutritional deficiency and confirming the benefit of cod liver oil.

The surprise was that, beginning in the spring, the Pirquet babies with rickets began to improve with no change in their diet. By the middle of the summer, all the children were growing healthy bones. Diet seemed to matter only in the winter.

The women were perplexed. Holding to their nutritional theory, they explored the possibility that it was the dairy cows' diet that mattered. Perhaps cows in the summer ate better feed and produced more nutritious milk than in the winter. However, they found that the cows were all stall-fed on the same feed year-round. Margaret Hume, believing the anti-rachitic substance was fat-soluble A, tested milk for its ability to support the growth of young rats, the standard biological assay for fat-soluble A. She found that the milk was equally, although poorly, effective throughout the year.

The Lister Institute investigators then became aware of a publication by Kurt Huldschinsky, a Berlin physician, reporting that he had cured rickets by exposing children to ultraviolet light from a mercury vapor lamp.[5] The investigators then "knew that early spring sunshine on open verandahs had betrayed us" and designed a second experiment to explain why all the children got better in the summer.[6]

During the second year of the study, they studied children admitted during the winter with established rickets. They gave all the children Diet I and compared three additional treatments: cod liver oil, exposure to ultraviolet light from a mercury vapor lamp, and exposure to outdoor sunlight. The first two groups remained indoors in a ward brightly sunlit, but through glass windows that blocked ultraviolet light.

All the children improved. Three who were both exposed to outdoor sunlight and given cod liver oil improved most rapidly. By the middle of the summer, they were all growing healthy bones. Either cod liver oil or ultraviolet light could cure rickets. The investigators also made the important observation that if only one leg of a rachitic child was exposed to ultraviolet light from the mercury vapor lamp, all their limbs improved equally. The effect was systemic, not just local.

The investigators reported their results in a 1922 paper in *The Lancet*.[7] They took the opportunity to point out the mistaken conclusions of their rivals in Glasgow, who had aggressively argued that the cause of rickets was a lack of exercise and fresh air, dismissing the importance of nutrition and ignoring the role of sunlight. Harriette Chick and her coworkers did not understand the mechanism, but they had explained the observations of the Glasgow group by demonstrating the benefit of ultraviolet light, either from a lamp or from the sun. They drove their point home in their paper. "We have obtained no evidence that fresh air or exercise produced any effect apart from the concomitant greater incidence of sunlight, and our observations, we think, prove that, with a minimal isolation, as during winter, diet is the controlling factor."

One of the Glasgow workers, Dr. Lionel Findlay, had visited Vienna to observe the rickets studies. He had been "captious and argumentative" according to Harriette.[8] It must have felt good to put him in his place.

With the new observations of the benefit of ultraviolet light, the Lister Institute investigators modified their ideas about the role of nutrition. They admitted their error in equating rickets with scurvy and beriberi and ascribing it solely to a deficient diet. They now recognized that "a faulty diet, if operating at all, is not the sole factor." But diet was one factor. Babies who did not obtain sufficient vitamin D in their diets were at risk for developing rickets when kept indoors out of the sun during the winter. Superimposed on a diet deficient in animal fats, the amount of sun exposure became the major determinant of who would get the disease. This explained the seasonal variation in incidence as well as the prevalence in smoggy industrial cities.

Although the Lister Institute investigators revised their views regarding the role of diet in the etiology of rickets, they held to their belief in the role of vitamins. They speculated that ultraviolet light induced the synthesis of the same vitamin supplied by cod liver oil, a speculation soon proved correct by other investigators.

Adult Bones Also Suffered

Adults shared with children the same lack of animal fats in the diet and infrequent sun exposure during the winter. Consequently, they also suffered vitamin D deficiency. This produced an inability to absorb calcium from the intestine and low blood calcium. The bones lost minerals, became brittle, fractured easily, and were painful. The condition was termed *hunger osteomalacia*. Physicians recognized its relation to rickets: the two diseases occurred in the same geographical areas, and both were worse in late winter and spring and tended to remit during the summer. The condition was most common in the elderly, presumably because they spent less time outdoors than younger people.

By the end of the war, hunger osteomalacia had become common in Vienna, especially among the poor. It was a particular problem in convents, where access to food was limited both by the pervading shortages and by the hostility of the government to the Catholic Church. In addition, many of the sisters got little outdoor exercise, spending virtually all year indoors. Harriette wrote to Charles Martin that "The places are dark and cold and give you what Dr. Dalyell calls 'the croodles.'"[9] Consequently, both younger and older nuns suffered, and they suffered year-round.

In their 1921 paper in *The Lancet,* Elsie Dalyell and Harriette Chick described the clinical features of the disease and reported the results of an uncontrolled clinical trial. To test their theory that hunger osteomalacia was caused by a faulty diet, they studied the effect of dietary supplements in 39 cases, 21 nuns in an Ursaline convent and 18 hospitalized patients with severe disease.[10] The Society of Friends Emergency Committee provided the extra foods to be added to the patients' ordinary diet, "which was always deficient in fat and always scanty." Merely providing added calories with sugar or cereal was of little benefit; but added fat (butter, margarine, olive oil or cod liver oil) produced recoveries. Cod liver oil was the most beneficial. In some of the nuns, who began the study bedridden, "the effect of cod liver oil seemed miraculous."[11]

In a companion paper, Margaret Hume, along with a Viennese physician, Edmund Nirenstein, reported a test of cod liver oil in 130 outpatients of a medical relief clinic.[12] They compared the standard treatment at the time, a mixture of phosphorus in vegetable oil*, to cod liver oil in a controlled trial of 131 patients. The cod liver oil proved markedly superior.

The efficacy of cod liver oil in treating both rickets and hunger osteomalacia strengthened the presumed relationship between the two diseases. And yet another disease was shown to be treatable with dietary manipulations.

Mission Accomplished

Harriette and her colleagues had reconciled the two main theories of rickets. Rickets could be prevented or cured either through a diet enriched in animal fats or through exposure to ultraviolet light. Presumably both treatments provided the same vitamin. Although dietary animal fats contained that nutrient, the lack of sunlight, superimposed on a poor diet, was the main cause of the epidemics of rickets in northern industrial cities.

Both human breast milk and cows' milk are poor sources of vitamin D; but children in the country spent time in the sun and avoided the disease, while those in industrial cities darkened by air pollution suffered vitamin D deficiency. At the same time the work in Vienna was being carried out, Alfred Hess in New York confirmed the benefit of sunlight in yet another city with gray skies.[13]

Over the next decade, scientists in Europe and the United States worked out the physiology. Vitamin D was distinguished from vitamin A and earned its own name. Chemists found a family of related molecules sharing vitamin D activity and Adolf Otto Reinhold Windaus won the Nobel Prize in 1928 for determining their chemical structures. Others elucidated the role of ultraviolet light in inducing their synthesis in the skin. The various forms of vitamin D were synthesized in the laboratory, produced in factories and added to milk and to the diet of nursing mothers.

---

* A preparation called Phosphor Öl.

The English disease did not disappear entirely but became uncommon in the developed world. The downside was that children the world over had cod liver oil forced upon them, whether they needed it or not. A friend of mine who grew up in rural Australia, where she was bathed with plenty of sunlight, wrote:

My Father knew about cod liver oil! Born in 1900 in the slums of Liverpool he and his siblings scavenged for food. In 1908 he was sent to an orphanage after his mother and brother died in the work house. He couldn't believe his luck, food and an opportunity to go to school. It was here that he was given a regular dose of cod liver oil. Many years later living in a remote part of rural Victoria (Australia that is), I too was given a weekly dose of cod liver oil. The hideous muck delivered on a spoon was followed by a teaspoon of jam. It's impossible to describe the trauma of this weekly event. Returning to a more civilized community and access to reasonable food brought it to an end, (more or less), but the aversion remains.[14]

Another friend, who grew up in Germany, was treated even worse. She was given only matzah crackers as a chaser.[15]

The Lister Institute team was proud of its contribution to public health. "It was no longer necessary for stunted and bowlegged men to be seen every day in the streets."[16] However, nothing the women demonstrated in Vienna was novel. Others had reported the benefit of cod liver oil, ultraviolet light and sunlight in animals and in uncontrolled observations in children. Nevertheless, these scattered reports had failed to convince the medical community.

The contribution of Chick and her colleagues was to prove those benefits by taking advantage of a unique environment in which to conduct carefully designed and well-documented controlled clinical trials. The combination of widespread infant malnutrition and the services of the Kinderklinik did not exist anywhere else in the world. Their paper in *The Lancet* left no doubts about their conclusions. In Harriette Chick's words:

Controls were only too abundant and we were regarded, possibly with some suspicion, as experimenters who were foolish enough to study the effects of additions to diets which local scientific and medical opinion regarded as quantitatively adequate. This being so, our trials were controlled in an unusually perfect manner and we were enabled to obtain a vindication of our theories which proved convincing to the most skeptical.[17]

In going to Vienna at the end of World War I, Harriette Chick once again was at the right place at the right time. More importantly, she had the courage, drive, and intelligence to take advantage of the opportunity. These studies established Harriette Chick as one of the most important medical researchers of her day. She returned to London in 1922 to resume her laboratory research, a mature scientist with a record of scientific productivity rivaling that of her most accomplished colleagues.

Notes

1   Chick H, Dalyell EJ (1921) Observations on the influence of foods rich in accessory factors in stimulating development in backward children. *Br Med J* 2 (3182) 1061-1066.

2   Chick H, Dalyell EJ, Hume M, Mackay HMM, Henderson Smith H, Wimberger H (1922) The etiology of rickets in infants: prophylactic and curative observations at the Vienna University Kinderklinik. *Lancet* 200 (5157) 7-11.

3   Mackay HMM (1920) Observation on cases of rickets in an out-patient department. *Br Med J* 2 (3129): 929-932.

4   Chick, Harriette; Margaret Hume; Marjorie Macfarlane. *War on Disease. A History of the Lister Institute* (London: Andre Deutsch, 1971), p. 158.

5   Huldschinsky K (1919) Heilung von Rachitis durch Küntlich Höhensonne. *Deutsh Med Woch* 45: 712-713.

6   Hume EMM (1944) Opportunities for nutritional research in the work of relief. *Proc Nutr Soc* 2 (3-4) 204-210.

7   Chick H, Dalyell EJ, Hume M, Mackay HM, Henderson Smith H, Wimberger H (1922) The etiology of rickets in infants: prophylactic and curative observations at the Vienna University Kinderklinik. *Lancet* 200 (5157): 7-11

8   Quoted by Carpenter KJ (2008) Harriette Chick and the problem of rickets. *J Nutrition* 138 (5): 827-832.

9   Extract of a letter from Miss Chick to Dr. Martin dated 1 January, 1920. National Archives of Great Britain.

10 Dalyell EJ, Chick H (1921) Hunger-osteomalacia in Vienna, 1920. I. Its relation to diet. *Lancet* 198 (5121): 842-849.

11 Chick H (1945) Nutritional researches in Vienna after the First World War. *Proc Nutrition Soc* 3 (1): 59-67.

12 Hume ME, Nirenstein E (1921) II. Comparative treatment of cases of hunger-osteo-malacia in Vienna, 1920, as out-patients with cod-liver oil and plant oil. *Lancet* 198 (5121): 849- 853.

13 Hess AF, Unger LJ (1921) The cure of infantile rickets by sunlight. *J Amer Med Assn* 77: 39-41

14 Helme, Beryl, personal communication, February 26, 2022.

15 Iris, Cristen, personal communication, February 25, 2024.

16 Chick H et al. (1975) *War on Disease*, p. 160.

17 Chick H (1945) Nutritional researches in Vienna after the First World War. *Proc Nutrition Soc* 3 (1): 59-67

CHAPTER 9
RE-ENTRY

In 1922, Harriette Chick, then forty-seven years old, returned to London and moved back in with her family in Ealing. It must have been a jolt to return to family life in a quiet neighborhood on the outskirts of London after living independently in cosmopolitan Vienna.

And she returned to a country where women were forced back into their traditional roles. Women had kept the economy going while men were away at war; but when the men returned, they resumed their jobs and the women were demoted or dismissed. In 1918, the final year of the war, fourteen of thirty scientific staff of the Lister Institute were women.[1] Two years later, only four remained, one listed as honorary and one as temporary.[2] Only Harriette Chick and Muriel Robertson remained on the active staff. Many women married and, whether they wanted to or not, gave up their careers since married women were generally excluded from professional positions.

Harriette never married. She left no record of whether she saw this as a sacrifice to do her duty to science, if she found science so engaging that she preferred a career to a family, or if she had no interest in having a family of her own. In her era, she could not have had the success she enjoyed professionally if she had married. As described by Kate Zernike in her book *The Exceptions* and documented systematically by Claudia Goldin, the winner of the 2023 Nobel Prize in Economics, the conflict between career and marriage continues until the present day.[3]

While Harriette went back to laboratory work, the clinicians on the Vienna team went their separate ways. Helen Mackay built a career as an academic pediatrician and became a leading expert on childhood nutrition and iron deficiency anemia. In 1934, she was the first woman elected to the Royal College of Physicians.

Elsie Dalyell was less successful. She went home to Australia, taking the opportunity to make a speaking tour of major universities of the United States and Canada on her way. Once back in Australia, she faced the same barriers as women in the United Kingdom. She was denied an appointment to a hospital staff and an attempt at a private practice was unsuccessful. After working for the Department of Public Health for three years, she, along with a colleague, opened a venereal disease clinic for women in suburban Sydney. Long before the invention of antibiotics, she could offer little effective treatment.

Back in the Laboratory

Having responded to the demands of the war and its aftermath, Harriette was free to choose the direction of her research. Rather than return to bacteriology, she continued to study nutrition. It remained a fertile area of investigation and her work in Vienna had cemented her place as a leading investigator in the field. Moreover, she could be the head of the Lister Institute nutrition program rather than being just one of many investigators studying infectious diseases.

However, she got off to a slow start. Prior to going to Vienna, Harriette had made her laboratory the best in the world at studying nutrition using biological assays in whole animals. The meticulous attention she and her coworkers devoted to caring for the animals and maintaining tight control over the experimental protocol were unrivaled. But the experiments were tedious, time-consuming, and labor-intensive. The animals had to be weighed and examined periodically for weeks, even months. Frequently, they had to be hand-fed. Uneaten food was collected daily. Feces were collected, weighed, and sometimes chemically analyzed. One experiment could take a year or more. This was a slow and demanding path to discovery.

On returning to London, Harriette had to restart a research program that had been dormant for three years, teaching new personnel the biological assays. Harriette knew these methods well but they were challenging for the neophyte. And Harriette Chick had high standards. Furthermore, as head of an expanded Nutrition Division, much of her time was occupied with administration. The National Archives of Great Britain contains numerous letters, many hand-written, from Harriette Chick to Lister Institute and MRC administrators justifying even modest expenditures. The letters are written in bureaucratic style and signed "Believe me. Harriette Chick."

Readjustment to life in London, lingering post-war disruption of operations at the Lister Institute, and fatigue after a demanding stint in Vienna may have all played a part in limiting her productivity. The prevailing sexism undoubtedly deterred men from subordinating themselves to a female laboratory chief, making it difficult for her to recruit personnel. Her main coworkers over the next decade were women, Margaret Roscoe, Alice Copping, and Margaret Boas.

Harriette's only publications over the next three years were studies refining the experiments she and Margaret Hume had begun in Vienna on the influence of the diet of cows on the anti-rachitic activity of milk.[4] They had assumed that the anti-rachitic substance was vitamin A, the fat-soluble substance discovered by E. V. McCollum necessary for the normal growth of young rats; and Margaret Hume had shown that the vitamin A content of milk was constant year-round. However, McCollum and others had found that the anti-rachitic vitamin was distinct from vitamin A and, consistent with Hume's work, that the cow's diet did not affect the vitamin A content of its milk.[5] Now knowing that the anti-rachitic substance was not vitamin A, Harriette readdressed the issue of whether the conditions under which cows were housed and fed affected the anti-rachitic activity of the milk.

For these experiments she collaborated with Margaret Averil Boas, who at the time was a trainee in Martin's laboratory supported by the Grocers' Company.[*] The women used calcium and phosphorus retention in growing rats as a direct measure of anti-rachitic activity. They confirmed that the cow's

---

[*] The Worshipful Company of Grocers was founded in the 14th century as a guild of London grocers and evolved into a charitable institution known as the Grocers' Company. Margaret Averil Boas continued on as a biochemist at the Lister Institute and did work leading to the discovery of biotin (vitamin B7).

diet does not affect the anti-rachitic activity of its milk and published their findings in 1924 in the *Biochemical Journal.* [6]

Chick's productivity increased in 1926 with the publication of five papers in the *Biochemical Journal.* Three, co-authored with Margaret Roscoe, dealt with rickets. The first was a description of a model of rickets in young rats.[7] The second study used this model to confirm McCollum's observation that fat-soluble vitamin A and the anti-rachitic vitamin were distinct and to verify the lack of effect of diet and sunlight on the anti-rachitic activity of cows' milk.[8] The third paper demonstrated that spinach is a rich source of fat-soluble A but lacks vitamin D.[9] (By then, the anti-rachitic vitamin had acquired its permanent name.) The two other papers were purely methodological.[10]

These publications were merely confirmatory of prior results and added little to the understanding of rickets. Harriette Chick published no more original work on that disease, although she published a review article about ultraviolet light[11] and an original article concerning *fagopyrism*, photosensitivity in farm animals caused by a porphyrin in buckwheat.[12] She also wrote reviews of her work in Vienna.[13] The last of these was prepared for an oral presentation that she introduced in person two weeks before her hundredth birthday.[14]

Hunting for More Vitamins

Although Harriette did no more studies of rickets, she continued to focus on vitamins. A major unanswered question was: how many vitamins were there? Only four were known for certain:

- Vitamin B1, the anti-neuritic vitamin, the water-soluble substance in yeast and in the germ of grains that prevents beriberi.
- Vitamin C, the antiscorbutic vitamin, the water-soluble substance in fresh fruits and vegetables that prevents scurvy.
- Vitamin A (formerly fat-soluble A), the substance in butterfat and egg yolk necessary for the growth of young rats.
- Vitamin D, the anti-rachitic substance.

However, accumulating evidence indicated that there were more yet waiting to be discovered.

Chick's regular publications resumed in 1927 with a series of papers in which she attempted to tease out additional water-soluble vitamins, collectively called B vitamins. A motivation for these studies was the disease pellagra, which had become a prime candidate to join the list of vitamin deficiency diseases. Pellagra was a debilitating disease that became common in southern Europe during the eighteenth and nineteenth centuries and in the southeast of the United States during the twentieth. It had a complicated history and complicated biochemistry that baffled scientists. And Harriette was as baffled as the rest.

Pellagra, the Red Evil

Pellagra typically begins with sores in the mouth, making eating painful. This is followed by red, dry, fissured skin, especially in sun-exposed areas, and by diarrhea and neuropsychiatric symptoms. The mnemonic taught to medical students is *the three D's*: dermatitis, diarrhea, and dementia. Some add a fourth D, death, since the disease was frequently fatal. It is now rare in the developed world but continues to occur in sub-Saharan Africa.

Don Gaspar Casal, a Spanish court physician, is credited with the first description of the disease in the medical literature. He described cases he saw during his thirty-three years practicing medicine in Asturias, where the disease was called *mal de la rosa* (the red evil) because of the characteristic red rash. Although his cases dated from as early as 1735, his work was only published posthumously in 1762. [15] In 1771, the Italian physician Francesco Frapolli introduced the term *pellagra* (rough skin), the name for the disease employed by peasants in Lombardy. [16] Over the next century, the disease became common in southern Europe, the Balkans, Egypt and other parts of Africa.

Casals and other early observers recognized that pellagra was associated with corn and poverty.[17] After Christopher Columbus brought corn from the Americas to Europe, it rapidly became the predominant crop in areas surrounding the Mediterranean Sea, where land planted in corn was more productive than that planted with wheat or barley. For impoverished peasants, boiled corn and cornmeal came to be staples of their diet and an epidemic of pellagra ensued. The disease was blamed on the consumption of spoiled, contaminated corn. The belief was that the corn either contained a toxin or transmitted an infection. The association with poverty was attributed to the poor having to make do with spoiled corn, while the rich could throw out the old and buy fresh.

Pellagra in fact results from a dietary deficiency of niacin (vitamin B3, either nicotinic acid or nicotinamide); but the biochemistry is complex, which delayed understanding the disease.[18] The recognition in 1917 that a disease of dogs, called *black tongue*, was the canine equivalent of pellagra hastened progress.[19] Nevertheless, it was not until 1935 that Conrad A. Elvehjem and Carl J. Koehn, Jr., at the University of Wisconsin, chemically separated the substance that prevented pellagra from other B vitamins.[20] They went on to identify it as niacin.[21]

As well as being available from many foods—especially meat, fish and legumes—niacin can be synthesized from the essential amino acid trypto-phan, so that a diet high in tryptophan or in proteins that contain tryptophan can prevent pellagra when the diet is deficient in niacin. However, zein, the major protein in corn, lacks tryptophan. Moreover, although corn kernels contain niacin, it is bound to a starch, hemicellulose, and is not absorbed from the intestine. In Europe and Africa, the practice was to boil corn kernels in water to soften them and make them palatable. This does not release the niacin. Too poor to supplement their diet with other sources of niacin, the peasants suffered from pellagra.

However, peoples of Mexico and Central and South America, who had depended for centuries on corn as a dietary staple, did not suffer from the dis-ease. They prepared corn dough, *masa*, by boiling the kernels in an alkaline solution, a process termed *nixtamalization*. This not only softens the kernels, but also releases the niacin so that it can be absorbed. Plus, they included beans in their diet, providing both tryptophan and niacin. If the conquista-dors had stolen the recipes of the indigenous people of the Americas along with their gold, thousands of European lives would have been saved.

Pellagra did not become prevalent in the United States until the begin-ning of the twentieth century, when it became epidemic in textile mill towns in the South. In Harriette Chicks words, "the disease seems to stand in much the same relationship with the eating of maize as beriberi stands with the eating of rice."[22] Like beriberi, the epidemic of pellagra in the United States was the result of new milling technology.

Impoverished farm and cotton mill workers and their families subsisted on a diet of cornbread, grits (cornmeal), molasses, and some meat, principally fatback since it was cheap.[23] In rural areas, people grew their own corn and milled it by hand. They also included other vegetables in their diet, protecting them from pellagra. However, the invention of the Beall degerminator in 1901 permitted the industrial production of cornmeal. People living in the mill towns, which were served by railroads, did not grow and mill their own corn but made their cornbread and grits from cornmeal shipped from factories in the Midwest and sold in company stores.

Unlike hand milling, the industrial process removed the germ from the corn kernels. That extended the shelf life of the cornmeal and made its transportation over long distances feasible; but it also removed much of the niacin. Moreover, the diet of families in the towns was more restricted than in rural areas. The result was an epidemic of pellagra in southern states that began during the first decade of the twentieth century and extended through the 1930s. Over that time, the disease affected over three million people and killed over 100,000.

Joseph Goldberger was the investigator who made the biggest contribution to understanding this epidemic.[24] He was born in a village in what is now Slovakia. When he was nine years old, his family immigrated to the United States, where he grew up on the Lower East Side of Manhattan, giving him empathy for the impoverished. He was a talented student and obtained his medical education at Bellevue Hospital, whose medical school accepted Jewish immigrants.

After graduation and a brief period of private practice, Goldberger joined the United States Public Health Service. He began that career by traveling through the southern United States and Mexico investigating epidemics of infectious diseases, his travels punctuated by periods of laboratory research in Washington, DC. His intelligence and diligence impressed his supervisors.

In 1914, responding to pressure from Congress, the Surgeon General initiated an investigation of the pellagra epidemic. A committee of experts, the Thompson-McFadden Commission, citing an epidemiological survey of households near Spartanburg, South Carolina, had concluded that pellagra was a contagious disease.[25] Goldberger was the ideal person to track down the cause of the infection and the Surgeon General asked him to lead the effort.

However, Goldberger quickly realized that the Commission's conclusion was wrong. He noted that in chronic-care hospitals pellagra was common among the patients but never occurred among the staff, many of whom lived in the institutions, some in the same wards as the patients, having close, daily contact with them over a period of years.[26] Goldberger asked, "If pellagra be a communicable disease, why should there be this exemption of the nurses and attendants?" His answer was that the diets of the two groups differed. Although the staff ate with the patients in a common dining room, they got the first pick of the food and supplemented their institutional diet with more varied fare.[27]

As early as 1912, Casimer Funk had hypothesized that pellagra was a vitamin deficiency disease and suggested that it was related to the industrial milling of corn.[28] Goldberger agreed that the cause was a faulty diet, but initially made the wrong assumption about what was missing, thinking it was animal protein. Nevertheless, he conducted three experiments that confirmed that the disease was nutritional. In two experiments, he added meat, milk, and beans to the diets of groups of residents of institutions with a high prevalence of pellagra. The patients receiving the enriched diets were protected from the disease.[29]

For the third experiment, Goldberger did the opposite: he took food away from healthy men. He conducted his experiment at the Rankin Prison Farm, near Jackson, Mississippi, then a state prison for white men.* The inmates enjoyed a varied diet that included meat, milk, peas, and beans; and none suffered from pellagra.[30] To induce prisoners to volunteer, Goldberger persuaded Governor Earl Brewer to offer pardons to those who served as experimental subjects.

Goldberger enrolled twelve healthy men. He separated them from the other inmates and fed them a diet containing mainly cornbread, grits, gravy, and syrup. After five months on the restricted diet, six men showed signs of pellagra. Goldberger invited experienced physicians to examine the men and they independently confirmed his diagnoses. No other inmates of the prison developed the disease. Goldberger thought he had proven the nutritional

* Now the site of the Central Mississippi Correctional Facility.

cause of pellagra and vigorously advocated for improvements in the diet of impoverished Southerners.

But the Rankin Prison Farm experiment did not convince everyone. Critics refused to accept that pellagra was other than an infection that resulted from inadequate hygiene among the poor and was in part their own fault. The skeptics either called into question the diagnosis of pellagra among the volunteers in Goldberger's experiment or maintained that he had starved them, weakening their immune system and making them susceptible to a chronic infection. Moreover, the ethics of using prisoners as experimental subjects and of pardoning convicted criminals generated controversy.

Pellagra became a hot-button political issue.[31] Southern politicians bristled at the suggestion that there was widespread malnutrition in their region, with the implication that the South remained economically undeveloped. The party line was that the New South had risen from the ashes of the Civil War, had industrialized with the growth of textile manufacturing, and was no longer a backwards agricultural economy. In fact, pellagra disproportionately affected the mill towns created by that industrialization; and Goldberger had called the party line into question.

He was criticized by many Southern physicians. He was accused of being biased, even of faking the Rankin Prison Farm experiment.[32] But Goldberger was a bulldog. He had dedicated his life to the public health and he was confident of his science. He persisted in advocating for improvements in the diet of impoverished millworkers and continued to study pellagra. In his laboratory studies, he came around to the vitamin deficiency camp and tried to isolate the *pellagra-preventative factor* (P-P factor), as he termed it. These studies came to a premature end when he died in 1929 at the age of fifty-five.

Mistaken Assumptions and Slow Progress

Harriette Chick was convinced that pellagra was a nutritional deficiency disease. In 1920, she published a paper reporting her attempt to produce pellagra in three monkeys by administering a protein-deficient diet, testing Goldberger's original hypothesis that the missing nutrient in the pellagrous diet was animal protein. Although she tried to make the case that a rash on the monkeys' faces resembled that of pellagra, in fact, she had only produced protein deficiency and general malnutrition.[33] She did not resume her study of pellagra until later in the decade, when it was apparent that the missing nutrient was an unknown vitamin.

Beginning in 1927, Harriette Chick and Margaret Roscoe published three papers that reported their first attempts to find what was missing in the diet of pellagra sufferers by looking for water-soluble vitamins, B vitamins, in addition to the anti-neuritic substance.* This entailed developing chemical methods to isolate individual micronutrients from yeast extract. They began by separating the anti-neuritic vitamin from a water-soluble substance that promoted the growth of young rats, mistakenly assuming that this was the same as the substance that prevented pellagra, Goldberger's P-P factor.

The only method Chick and Roscoe had to detect the nutrients was biological assays. However, they had no way of knowing that the use of rats for these assays was a fatal flaw. They knew that, unlike birds which develop nerve degeneration identical to that of beriberi when deprived of thiamin, rats deprived of the vitamin die before developing nerve degeneration. Chick and Roscoe tried to get around this problem by developing an assay based on the growth of young rats, but this was not specific for vitamin B1 and could give misleading results.[34]

In addition, the women made sure the rats' diet contained abundant protein. It was not known at the time that the animals could synthesize niacin from tryptophan supplied by the protein. Furthermore, the women thought that skin changes in malnourished rats was the rodent equivalent of the rash of pellagra. In fact, skin changes are a consequence of deficiency of any of several B vitamins and not specific to niacin deficiency, a phenomenon Harriette later recognized and studied.[35]

Despite the limitations of their experimental design, the women made progress. They began with the conservative assumption that there were only two B vitamins: the anti-neuritic vitamin that prevented and cured beriberi, vitamin B1, and another substance that supported the growth of young rats, which Harriette called vitamin B2.† They developed methods to separate the

* Eight B vitamins are now recognized.

† In current nomenclature, vitamin B2 is reserved for riboflavin and the P-P factor, niacin, is vitamin B3.

two. A key aspect of their methods was that yeast extract lost its anti-neuritic activity when subjected to prolonged autoclaving at 120 C, whereas
the growth-promoting factor survived that treatment. In reality, both the
heat-stable and heat-labile fractions contained multiple B vitamins.

Subsequent papers refined the methods and explored the chemistry
of the B vitamins. [36] Of note, in the title of one paper published in 1930,
"anti-pellegra" appears in quotation marks, indicating doubt as to whether
the dermatitis they were producing in rats was the equivalent of human
pellagra. In 1930, Alice Copping joined the team. The three women
co-authored a paper reporting that egg white was a good source of the
growth-promoting B vitamin.[37] This study may have sprung from the independent work of Margaret Boas that eventually led to the isolation of biotin
(vitamin B7).[38]

By late 1930, Harriette Chick was convinced that her heat-stable fraction
contained more than one vitamin. She and Alice Copping titled a paper "The
composite nature of the water-soluble vitamin B" and subtitled it "Dietary
factors in addition to the anti-neuritic vitamin B(1) and the anti-dermatitis
vitamin B(2)."[39] But they did not know how many additional vitamins there
were nor their chemical nature, just that young rats required multiple substances in yeast extracts in addition to the anti-neuritic substance to grow
and remain healthy.

Although Chick, Roscoe, and Copping failed to find the vitamin missing
in pellagra sufferers, they verified the existence of multiple B vitamins and
helped motivate the chemists to purify and characterize them.

A Royal Honor

1932 was a banner year for Harriette. King George V awarded her the title
of Commander of the Most Excellent Order of the British Empire (C.B.E.),
which recognizes public service, including major contributions to the arts
and sciences. Whether by personal choice or as required by journals' style
manuals, the only later publications in which the suffix C.B.E. was affixed to
her name were in *Lancet*. She signed her other papers Harriette Chick, Lister
Institute of Preventive Medicine. Apparently, she was at least as proud of her
association with the Lister Institute as of royal titles.

As a further capstone to this phase of her career, Harriette made a speaking tour of the United States to describe her own work and to support Goldberger's nutritional explanation for pellagra.* She turned this into a round-the-world trip, visiting Charles Martin, who was working in Adelaide at the time, as well as other friends and colleagues.

A Change of Direction

Harriette eventually recognized that rats had been a poor choice for her experiments. She began a 1937 paper by stating "While the rat has been used in recent years with great success in nutritional studies, the results obtained have proved to be misleading in the investigation of pellagra."[40] She therefore turned to pigs to identify the P-P factor.

Local regulations prevented housing pigs in Chelsea, so Charles Martin, who by this time had retired to Cambridge, volunteered to care for them. Harriette and a colleague, Thomas F. Macrae, prepared the concentrated vitamins in London for Martin to feed to the pigs in Cambridge. However, the Lister team was soon scooped by Elvehjem and Koehn, who identified the P-P factor as niacin. They performed their biological assays in dogs, which, when fed a maize diet, develop black tongue disease, the canine equivalent of pellagra. In the end, Harriette's pig experiments merely confirmed the findings of Elvehjem and Koehn.[41] She published an additional paper in which she demonstrated that pigs required at least one B vitamin in addition to the anti-neuritic vitamin, nicotinic acid and riboflavin; but she did not follow this up and try to identify the essential nutrient.[42]

This line of Harriette's research—using whole-animal experiments to discover new vitamins—came to an end. During the decade beginning in 1916, when she entered the field, it had been highly productive, adding to the understanding of essential micronutrients and saving thousands of lives. However, with advances in chemistry and in the understanding of cellular metabolism, the chemists took over and Harriette Chick made no further efforts to identify unknown nutrients. She was no longer on the cutting edge of scientific discovery.

Nevertheless, many questions about nutrition remained unanswered. As

---

* I have been unable to find a record of specific talks or a copy of her notes.

her vitamin work wound down, Harriette turned to the study of proteins. Because individual proteins differ in their content of essential amino acids, they vary in their ability to support the health of animals. Harriette and coworkers, primarily Margaret Averil Boas*, published a series of seven papers in the *Biochemical Journal* trying to quantify these differences.[43]

The papers were substantially methodological. For one of them, they measured the ability of the proteins to support the growth of weanling rats. They were unable to demonstrate marked differences in the nutritional value of wheat, maize, and milk proteins; and the papers produced no important new discoveries. But the study of the growth of weanling rats laid the foundation for the work that Harriette Chick was to carry out during World War II. That work would have a major impact on the diet of Great Britain, promoting the adoption of the National Loaf.

Notes

1   Bruce D (1919) *Report of the Governing Body* (London: The Lister Institute of Preventive Medicine), p. 3.

2   Bruce D (1921) *Report of the Governing Body* (London: The Lister Institute of Preventive Medicine), p. 3.

3   Zernike, Kate (2023) *The Exceptions. Nancy Hopkins, MIT, and the Fight for Women in Science.* New York: Scribner.

     Goldin, Claudia. (2021) *Career & Family. Women's Century-Long Journey toward Equity.* Princeton: Princeton University Press.

4   Boas MA, Chick H (1924) The influence of diet and management of the cow upon the deposition of calcium in rats receiving a daily ration of milk in their diet. *Biochem J* 18 (2): 433-447.

5   McCollum EV, Simmonds, N, Shipley PG, Park EA (1922) Studies on experimental rickets. Is there a substance other than fat-soluble A associated with certain fats which plays an important role in bone development? *J Biol Chem* 50 (1): 5-30.

     McCollum EV, Simmonds N, Becker JE, Shipley PG (1922) Studies on experimental rickets. An experimental demonstration of the existence of a vitamin which promotes calcium deposition. *J Biol Chem* 53 (2): 293 – 312.

6   Boas MA, Chick H (1924) The influence of diet and management of the cow upon the

---

* Her married name was Boas Fixen.

deposition of calcium in rats receiving a daily ration of milk in their diet. *Biochem J* 18(2): 433-447.

7   Chick H, Korenchevsky V, Roscoe MH (1926) The difference in chemical composition of the skeletons of young rats fed (1) on diets deprived of fat-soluble vitamins and (2) on a low phosphorous rachitic diet, compared with those of normally nourished animals of the same age. *Biochem J* 20 (3): 622-631.

8   Chick H, Roscoe MH (1926) Influence of diet and sunlight upon the amount of vitamin A and Vitamin D in the milk afforded by a cow. *Biochem J* 20 (3): 632-649.

9   Chick H, Roscoe, MH (1926) The anti-rachitic value of fresh spinach. *Biochem J* 20 (1): 137-152.

10   Henderson Smith H, Chick H (1926) Maintenance of a standardized breed of young rats for work upon fat-soluble vitamins, with particular reference to the endowment of the offspring. *Biochem J* 20 (1): 131-136.

     Chick H (1926) Sources of error in the technique employed for the biological assay of fat-soluble vitamins. *Biochem J* 20 (1): 119-130.

11   Chick H (1932) The relation of ultra-violet light to nutrition. *Lancet* 220 (5686): 377-384.

12   Chick H, Ellinger P (1941) The photosensitizing action of buckwheat (*Fagopyrum esculentum*). *J Physiol* 100 (2): 212-230.

13   Chick H (1945) Nutritional researches in Vienna after the First World War. *Proc Nutr Soc* 3 (1): 59-67.

14   Chick H (1976) Study of rickets in Vienna 1919-1922. *Med Hist* 20: 41-51.

15   Casal, Don Gaspar (1762) *Historia natural, y medica de el Principado de Asturias.* (Madrid: Martin) p. 327. [Published in English translation in Ralph H. Major, *Classic Descriptions of Disease, 3rd Ed.* (Springfield, IL: Charles C. Thomas, 1945), pp. 610-614.]

16   Major RH (1944) Don Gaspar Casal, Francois Thiery and pellagra. *Bull Hist Med* 16 (4): 351-361.

17   Carpenter, KJ. (1983) The relationship of pellagra to corn and the low availability of niacin in cereals. In: J. Mauron, ed., *Nutritional Adequacy, Nutrient Availability and Needs* (Basel: Birlhauser Verlag, 1983), pp. 197-222.

18   Carpenter KJ. (1983) The relationship of pellagra to corn and the low availability of niacin in cereals. In: J. Mauron, ed., *Nutritional Adequacy, Nutrient Availability and Needs* (Basel: Birlhauser Verlag, 1983), pp. 197-222.

19   Chittenden RH, Underhill, FP (1917) The production in dogs of a pathological condition which closely resembles human pellagra. *Proc Natl Acad Sci USA* 3 (3): 195-197.

20   Elvehjem CA, Koehn CJ, Jr., Oleson JJ (1936) A new essential dietary factor. *J Biol Chem* 115 (3): 707-719.

21   Elvehjem CA, Madden RJ, Strong FM, Woolley DW (1938) The isolation and identi-
      fication of the anti-black tongue factor. *J Biol Chem* 123 (1): 137-149.

22   Chick H, Hume EM (1920) The production in monkeys of symptoms closely resem-
      bling those of pellagra, by prolonged feeding on a diet of low protein content.
      Biochem J 14 (2): 135-146.

23   McCollum, Elmer Verner (1957) *A History of Nutrition* (Boston: Houghton Mifflin),
      pp. 302-318.

24   Kraut, Alan M. (2003) *Goldberger's War. The Life and Work of a Public Health
      Crusader.* New York: Hill and Wang.

25   Siler JF, Garrison PE, MacNeal WJ (1914) Pellagra: a summary of the first progress
      report of the Thompson-McFadden Pellagra Commission. *J Amer Med Assn* 62 (1):
      8 – 12.

26   Goldberger J (1914) The etiology of pellagra. The significance of certain epidemio-
      logical observations with respect thereto. *Public Health Rep* 29 (26): 1683-1686.

27   Goldberger J (1914) The etiology of pellagra. The significance of certain epidemio-
      logical observations with respect thereto. *Public Health Rep* 29 (26): 1683-1686.

28   Funk C (1912) The etiology of the deficiency diseases. Beri-beri, polyneuritis in
      birds, epidemic dropsy, scurvy, experimental scurvy in animals, infantile scurvy,
      ship beri-beri, pellagra. *J. State Med* 20:341-368. [Reprinted in Samuel A. Goldblith
      and Maynard A. Joslyn, eds., *Milestones in Nutrition* (Westport CT: Avi Publishing,
      1964), pp.145-172.]

      Funk, C. (1913) Studies on pellagra. I. The influence of the milling of maize on the
      chemical composition and the nutritive value on maize-meal. *J. Physiol* 47 (4-5):
      389-392.

29   Goldberger J, Waring CH (1915) The prevention of pellagra. A test of diet among
      institutional inmates. *Public Health Rep* 30 (43): 3117-3131.

      Goldberger J, Waring CH, Tanner WF (1923) Pellagra prevention by diet among
      institutional inmates. *Public Health Rep* 38 (41): 2361-2368.

30   Goldberger J, Wheeler GA (1915) Experimental pellagra in the human subject
      brought about by a restricted diet. *Public Health Rep* 30 (46): 3336-3339.

31   Bollett AJ (1992) Politics and pellagra: the epidemic of pellagra in the U.S. in the
      early twentieth century. *Yale J Biol Med* 65 (3): 211-221.

32   Kraut AM (2003) *Goldberger's War*, 144.

33   Chick H, Hume EM (1920) The production in monkeys of symptoms closely resem-
      bling those of pellagra by prolonged feeding on a a diet of low protein content.
      Biochem J 14 (2): 135 – 146.

34   Chick H, Roscoe MH (1929) A method for the assay of the antineuritic vitamin B_1, in
      which the growth of young rats is used as a criterion. *Biochem J* 23 (3): 498-503.

35   Chick H, Macrae TF, Worden AN (1940) Relation of skin lesions in the rat to defi-
     ciency in the diet of different B2-vitamins. *Biochem J* 34 (4): 580-594.

36   Chick H, Roscoe MH (1929) An attempt to separate vitamin B2 from vitamin B1 in
     yeast and a comparison of its properties with those of the antineuritic vitamin B1.
     Biochem J 23 (3): 504-513.

     Chick H (1929) The effect on vitamin B2 of treatment with nitrous acid. *Biochem J*
     23 (3): 514-516.

     Chick H, Roscoe MH (1930) Heat-stability of the (anti-dermatitis, "anti-pellagra")
     water-soluble vitamin B2. *Biochem J* 24 (1): 105-112.

     Chick H, Copping AM (1930) The alcohol-solubility of the anti-dermatitis, more
     heat-stable vitamin B2 constituent of the vitamin B complex. *Biochem J* 24 (6):
     1744-1747.

37   Chick H, Copping AM, Roscoe MH (1930) Egg-white as a source of the anti-derma-
     titis vitamin B(2). *Biochem J* 24 (6): 1748-1753.

38   Boas, M. A. (1927) The effect of desiccation upon the nutritive properties of egg-
     white. *Biochem J* 21 (3): 712-724.

39   Chick H, Copping HM (1930) The composite nature of the water-soluble vitamin B:
     Dietary factors in addition to the antineuritic vitamin B(1) and the anti-dermatitis
     vitamin B(2). *Biochem J* 24 (6): 1764-1769.

40   Birch TW, Chick H, Martin CJ (1937) Experiments with pigs on a pellagra-produc-
     ing diet. *Biochem J* 31 (11): 2065-2079.

41   Chick H, Macrae TF, Martin AJP, Martin CJ (1938) The curative action of nicotinic
     acid on pigs suffering from the effects of a diet consisting largely of maize. *Biochem
     J.* 32 (1): 10-12.

     Chick H, Macrae TF, Martin AJP, Martin CJ (1938) Experiments with pigs on a
     pellagra-producing diet. II. *Biochem J* 32 (5): 844-854.

42   Chick H, Macrae TF, Martin AJP, Martin CJ (1938c) The water-soluble B-vitamins
     other than aneurin (vitamin B(1)), riboflavin and nicotinic acid required by the pig.
     Biochem J 32 (12): 2207-2224.

43   Chick H, Roscoe MH (1930) The biological values of proteins. I. A method for mea-
     suring the nitrogenous exchange of rats for the purpose of determining the biological
     value of proteins. *Biochem J* 24 (6): 1780-1782.

     Boas Fixsen MA (1930) The biological values of proteins. II. The biological value of
     purified caseinogen and the influence of vitamin B2 upon biological values, deter-
     mined by the balance sheet method. *Biochem J* 24 (6): 1794-1804.

     Boas Fixsen MA, Jackson HM (1932) The biological values of proteins. III. A further
     note on the method used to measure the nitrogenous exchange of rats. *Biochem J* 26
     (6): 1919-1922.

     Boas Fixsen MA, Jackson HM (1932) The biological values of proteins. IV. The bio-
     logical values of the proteins of wheat, maize and milk. *Biochem J* 26 (6): 1923-1933.

Boas-Fixsen MA, Hutchinson JCD and Jackson HM (1934) The biological values of proteins. V. The comparative biological values of the proteins of whole wheat, whole maize and maize gluten, measured by the growth of young rats. *Biochem J* 28 (2): 592-601.

Chick H, Hutchinson JCD, Jackson HM (1935) The biological value of proteins. VI. Further investigation of the balance sheet method. *Biochem J* 29 (7): 1702-1711.

Chick H, Boas-Fixsen MA, Hutchinson JCD, Jackson HM (1935) The biological value of proteins. VII. The influence of variation in the level of protein in the diet and of heating the protein on its biological value. *Biochem J* 29 (7): 1712-1719.

CHAPTER 10

THE NATIONAL LOAF

Harriette continued doing in the laboratory what she did best, nutritional experiments in whole animals; but her career as an original investigator had peaked in Vienna. During the 1920s and 1930s, the major scientific advances came from the chemists and biochemists. She verified the work of others showing that there were B vitamins in addition to vitamin B1, but her attempts to identify those vitamins did not bear fruit.

As the scientific importance of her laboratory work waned, she took on more administrative responsibilities. In 1933, she was appointed to the Council of the Lister Institute, which functioned as a scientific advisory board to the Governing Body, the seven men who acted as the board of directors. She continued in the role, at least nominally, until 1975 when she was 100 years old. She also served on the League of Nations Committee on Nutrition from 1934 to 1937 and as Secretary of the MRC Accessory Food Factors Committee from its inception in 1918 until she retired in 1945. In addition, she was chair of the Committee on Vitamin Standards of the American Society of Biological Chemists.

In 1931 and 1934, the League of Nations convened meetings of its Permanent Commission on Biological Standardization. The Commission mandated studies on purified vitamin preparations to develop laboratory standards for their measurement. Harriette did her duty to science by accepting the mandate, but, as she noted in her annual progress report to Edward

Mellanby, then secretary of the MRC, these time-consuming studies occupied virtually all of Margaret Hume's time, taking her away from other work in the laboratory.[1]

As tensions built in Europe leading up to World War II, even more responsibilities demanded Harriette's time. Groups of nutrition scientists, mainly from London and Cambridge, met informally to discuss a food rationing system that could be put in place in case of war. Following on these meetings, a group of nutrition scientists, including Harriette Chick, Charles Martin and Edward Mellanby, in July 1941 proposed the organization of a Nutrition Society. Its main function would be to conduct meetings at which scientists from various disciplines could discuss the latest research related to human and animal nutrition.[2]

Harriette Chick served on the Executive Committee, which wrote by-laws, recruited members, and organized the initial scientific meetings. The committee met several times, culminating in the first scientific meeting of the Society in Cambridge in October 1941, and a second one at the London School of Hygiene and Tropical Medicine in February 1942. Because of the difficulties of wartime travel, a separate Scottish arm of the Society met at University College, Dundee. The Scots elected to maintain their separate identity after the War ended.

The initial meetings of both the English and Scottish divisions of the Society focused on supplying food to the British population during wartime. The topics included assessing the nutritional needs of humans and farm animals, organizing the food supply chain, and preventing waste. Because of the shortage of paper during the war, summaries of these meetings were not published until 1944, when permission was granted by the Paper Controller to print 1000 copies of the first issue of *Proceedings of the Nutrition Society*.[3]

With the outbreak of World War II in 1939, the Lister Institute relocated most of its work from Chelsea to outlying areas to escape the London Blitz. The Nutrition Department moved to Roebuck House, Dr. Martin's residence in Cambridge, which he leased from J. B. S. Haldane and to which he had retired in 1930. Harriette described it fondly:

The house had once been an inn and proved to be unusually well adapted for its new vocation. The spacious and well-heated conservatory made a famous animal house, an old coach house, affectionately known as the 'mediaeval lab,' was converted into a laboratory for rougher chemical work and preparation of food products, the workshop was pressed into service, and office and library accommodation was provided in the house proper. The necessary arrangements for water, gas and electricity were quickly made under the host's direction and largely with his own hands, in spite of his seventy odd years. A firm bench on which to stand fine balances was hard to arrange in so old a house, but a shelf was finally fixed in the wall of Martin's own room which in turn was invaded by the evacuees. Under these conditions more than five years were spent in happy and profitable work on vitamins and proteins. For finer chemical work a more suitable home was found at the Biochemical School [of Cambridge University] and for nutritional experiments with large animals at the Department of Animal Pathology. Roebuck House, however, remained the headquarters of the unit. Its host described himself as 'chief technical assistant,' was indeed all that and a very great deal more, for he was always at hand to share his invaluable experience and wise judgment and frequently to take a not inconsiderable part in the actual experiments.[4]

Harriette moved the laboratory animals from London to Cambridge in her family car.[5] However, she primarily remained in London, communicating by mail with Charles Martin, who supervised the work in Cambridge. Margaret Hume, Alice Copping, and Hannah Henderson Smith moved to Cambridge to conduct the animal experiments, which had been started by T. W. Birch, from the Cambridge University School of Veterinary Pathology.

The Bread Problem

As in World War I, Harriette Chick adapted her science to the demands of war. In contrast to World War I, when she focused on feeding the troops in the trenches, during World War II the challenge was feeding the civilians at home. Great Britain imported most of its food by sea, and German submarines torpedoed both military and commercial ships. From July through October of 1940, U-boats sank more than 280 Allied ships. Once Japan entered the war and occupied much of Southeast Asia, Pacific shipping came under attack and supplies of tea, sugar, rice, and spices were cut off.

The government reluctantly instituted food rationing and revived the Ministry of Food, first created during World War I. The British people, although with a lot of grumbling, accepted rationing as a fair system to distribute scarce resources.[6] The poor received the same rations as the rich, although the rich could more easily eat in clubs and restaurants. However, even restaurant meals were strictly regulated.

Bread was a special case. It accounted for 15% of the caloric intake of the average Englishman, and, as the cheapest source of calories, more than 30% for poor laborers and their families.[7] For the poor, an entire meal frequently consisted of "tea and two slices." Because of its importance in their diet, bread had a strong emotional quality for the British. It had not been rationed during the First World War; and Prime Minister Winston Churchill, fearing an effect on morale, refused to ration it during the Second.

Great Britain imported 70% of its wheat, mainly from Canada, but also from Australia, the United States, and Argentina. The wartime challenge was not only to decrease dependence of the food supply on risky transatlantic shipping but also to free up cargo space to transport war materials. The Ministry of Food tasked the MRC with finding ways to allow civilians to eat their fill of bread while minimizing the importation of wheat.

The MRC turned to the Accessory Food Factors Committee, of which Harriette was still secretary. The goal was to find ways to use wheat more efficiently and to optimize the nutritional value of flour. In principle, the solution to minimizing wheat importation was simple: use more of the wheat grain to make flour.

To make white flour, the wheat grain is milled and only the core—the *endosperm*—is retained. The milling removes the outer layer of bran, the aleurone layer which adheres to the bran, and the germ at the base of the grain—collectively termed the *offals*. The endosperm contains starch and the proteins that comprise gluten. In bread making, yeast metabolizes the starch and produces the carbon dioxide that makes bread rise.

This process of making white flour retains at most 75% of the grain, termed the *extraction percentage*. Dark brown, whole-grain flour, of 100% extraction, uses the entire grain. Intermediate grades of extraction retain variable amounts of bran and aleurone, either with or without the germ, and yield flours of different shades of brown.

Since ancient times, most people preferred white bread to brown.[8] Because producing white flour in stone mills was labor-intensive, throughout much of history it was more expensive than brown flour; and white bread was a luxury for the wealthy. Brown bread was food for the working people and, in the minds of the elite, associated with rural peasants.

In the middle of the nineteenth century, the tables turned. The development of steel roller milling machinery took the labor out of the production of white flour. Millers could then sell white flour to bakeries to make bread and pastries and gain additional income selling the offals to farmers for animal feed. Moreover, removing the germ made the flour keep better in storage. White flour became cheaper than brown and white bread became the staple of the working class. Brown bread became an affectation of the wealthy and of health enthusiasts advocating a return to the diet of the eighteenth-century rural farmer.

Through the second half of the nineteenth century and the first half of the twentieth, a debate raged about the relative nutritional value of white versus brown bread. And raged it did because the debate frequently became heated. It engaged economic self-interest on one side and deeply held beliefs about food on the other. Millers and bakers wanted to protect their income, while return-to-nature proponents advocated for whole-grain bread and a return to stone milling, ideally in wind-driven mills.

Sylvester Graham, a prominent nineteenth century activist, argued for a return to a pre-industrial lifestyle, including a diet of whole-grain bread and raw fruits and vegetables. Graham flour was his version of whole wheat flour and was the basis of Graham bread and Graham crackers, the same ones that are sold today. He wanted white flour banned and only whole-grain bread sold in bakeries. Another prominent voice was T. R. Allinson, who toured England preaching in favor of brown bread and vegetarianism and against vaccination. He was less extreme than Graham and allowed that people could cook their vegetables and live a modern lifestyle, gaining a wider audience as a result. The Bread and Food Reform League, formed in 1880, helped propagate these ideas.

The initial argument of the brown bread enthusiasts was that brown bread was more natural than white bread and provided more protein. After Eijkman's beriberi work became widely known, the preservation of vitamins in the germ and bran, especially vitamin B1, became an additional arm of their arguments. Without supporting evidence, they maintained that malnutrition, especially vitamin B1 deficiency, was common in England. They argued that poorly paid factory workers depended on bread and margarine for their calories and could not enjoy a varied diet to provide alternative sources of vitamins. Nutrition scientists generally sided with the brown bread activists, although the scientific basis of their arguments was weak.

The milling industry formed a powerful counterforce to the brown bread proponents. As business people, they wanted to provide the products the market desired. The millers were willing to fortify white flour with added vitamin B1 but strongly opposed being forced to produce brown flour. They would have to modify their milling machinery and would lose the income derived from selling the offals. They also argued for the benefits of degermination in extending the flour's shelf life.

The editorials in their magazine, *Milling*, were frequently combative, dismissing the nutritional activists as "fusspots" and pointing out the holes in their scientific arguments. Rats were not people, humans ate foods other than bread, and there was no convincing evidence that brown bread was more nutritious than fortified white bread. They also argued that the higher fiber content of brown bread might interfere with digestion.

The arguments of the brown bread advocates did not persuade many to change their eating habits. Immediately prior to World War II, 95% of the bread consumed in England was white, and efforts during the first months of the war to persuade shoppers to voluntarily change their buying patterns failed. A compulsory system had to be adopted. The challenge was to find a composition of flour that used more of the grain, that was at least as nutritious as unfortified white bread, and that was acceptable to consumers–or at least would not cause a popular uproar.

Harriette Chick entered the fray and became a prominent advocate for brown bread. She had begun studying the nutritional properties of bread in 1936 supported by the Millers' Association. Using the methods she had developed to study proteins, she compared the ability of various flours to support the growth of weanling rats. She first compared white flour supplemented with thiamine to wholemeal flour of 100% extraction.[9] Both groups of rats received casein to provide extra protein, cottonseed oil to provide lipids, cod liver oil to provide vitamins A and D, and a mixture of mineral salts. The rats fed the white flour grew at only about half the rate of the rats fed wholemeal flour. She summarized her conclusions:

> *The nutritive value of straight-run white flour* (73% extraction) tested*
> *on young growing rats, has been found inferior to that of wholemeal*
> *flour, even when the defects of the former in protein, minerals and vita-*
> *min B1 have been corrected. The inferiority must be attributed to the*
> *lack of B2 vitamins.*

The B2 vitamins, now termed vitamin B complex, were then known to include riboflavin and nicotinic acid, but also other uncharacterized essential nutrients.

Critics attacked her conclusions, mainly on the grounds that the rats fed the white flour ate less than the other group, hence obtained less protein.[10] They also questioned the relevance of weanling rats eating a restricted diet to humans eating a variety of foods. Nevertheless, her experiments were prominently cited in the debates over wartime bread.

Chick did further experiments to study proteins in the flours.[11] She compared wholemeal flour, wheatmeal flour of 85% extraction, and white flour, again measuring the growth of weanling rats. As in the prior experiments, she gave them cod liver oil to provide vitamins A and D. Unlike the prior experiment, she also gave them yeast extract to provide B vitamins. She therefore assumed that differences in growth would be a result of differences in the

---

* Straight-run flour was made by adjusting the milling machinery to produce a flour of the desired degree of extraction. The alternative was to add some of the bran back to white flour to achieve a similar composition.

proteins of the different flours. Here she expressed the results as *biological value*, the grams of weight gain per gram of protein ingested. The rats grew best on the wholemeal flour (biological value 1.6 to 1.77), less well on the wheatmeal flour (biological value 1.54 to 1.67) and least well on the white flour diet (biological value 1.21 to 1.48).

Harriette Chick conceded that "a 20% improvement in the biological value of the proteins of the bread eaten may not be important to a person eating a mixed diet in which the rest of the protein is provided by meat, milk, cheese and eggs." However, since few British civilians at that time took vitamin supplements, she surmised that "it is for the provision of B vitamins that the consumption of wholemeal flour, and of flours of higher degrees of extraction of the grain, is much more important." This conclusion may not have been firmly supported by her data but was not surprising from a scientist who had devoted her career to studying vitamins.

The other major workers on the bread problem were the team of Robert McCance and Elsie Widdowson, who spent their careers at King's College Hospital, London, studying nutrition. They did work similar to that of the Lister Institute workers and had a particular interest in mineral metabolism. Although the National Flour contained about twice as much calcium and phosphorus as white bread, it also contained almost four times as much phytic acid. McCance and Widdowson demonstrated that phytic acid binds phosphate and interferes with the intestinal absorption of both calcium and phosphorous.[12]

The brown bread advocates met with opposition from physicians as well as the milling industry. Some physicians argued that there was no evidence that the British population was deficient in vitamin B1, getting plenty from foods other than bread. Hence, its content in bread was irrelevant. Alternatively, thiamin could be produced commercially and added to white flour, the approach supported by the milling and baking industries.

Harriette Chick's experiments proved influential in the debate. Whether or not the English needed more thiamine, people required other vitamins and nutrients, some known and some unknown. Her demonstration that weanling rats grew better when fed brown rather than white bread, whether or not they were given yeast extract, persuaded many in Parliament. And Parliament had the final say.

Based on Harriette Chick's results and those of McCance and Widdowson, the MRC and the Accessory Food Factors Committee published two memos, one in May 1940 and the other in August 1941, detailing their recommended specifications for wheatmeal bread.[13] It was to be of 85% extraction, retain the germ, and discard as much of the bran as possible while retaining the aleurone layer, the outer coat of the endosperm which is rich in protein and vitamin B1. According to the MRC, of all the breads tested, 85% extraction flour "yielded the one which resembled white bread most closely in flavour and texture... The color of the bread was pale brown and was not unattractive."[14]

McCance and Widdowson's work with phytic acid led the MRC to recommend that the flour be fortified with calcium carbonate. The memos also specified that the flour not be bleached with oxidizing agents that would destroy its vitamins and that alkaline baking powders be avoided, as they would destroy the vitamin B1. They recommended against fortifying the flour with iron salts and against merely adding germ and some bran back to white flour.

The primary goal of the Ministry of Food was to reduce the importation of wheat and the MRC memos justified moving from white to brown bread. These arguments were mere political cover. Because of the savings in wheat, the Ministry would have adopted a high extraction flour as long as it was not nutritionally inferior to white bread.

The Ministry banned the sale of white bread as of April 6, 1942, and mandated that all bread sold in bakeries be the National Wheatmeal Loaf of 85% extraction.[15] In addition, the loaves had to be unsliced and unwrapped and could not be sold until at least a day old. The goal was to make the bread so unattractive to consumers that they would eat less of it. In a meeting of the Manchester District Master Bakers', Confectioners', and Caterers' Association, the president of the association said "that all efforts to make people eat wheatmeal bread had failed. Now, owing to the Government's order, they would have to eat it and it was the job of the bakers to make them like it."[16]

The bakers failed in that effort. With bran diluting the starch from the endosperm, the bread failed to rise properly, giving it a mushy consistency.

Many described its color as gray rather than light brown. It was called "Hitler's secret weapon." The National Loaf was not popular but it was all that was available.

The British accepted the need for sacrifice and wheatmeal bread became the staple. Even foreign dignitaries visiting Buckingham Palace were fed the National Loaf. The Government urged people to minimize bread consumption. Posters exhorted British civilians to "Eat Less Bread," to "Join the Crusade against the Waste of Bread," and to "Save a Loaf a Week—Help Win the War." One woman was fined £10 for feeding stale bread to birds. However, bread consumption increased by 30% over the course of the war, possibly because rationing restricted access to alternative foods.

Throughout the debate over the National Loaf, many nutrition scientists and activists went beyond the science to preach the benefits of brown bread. In her writings, Harriette Chick generally confined herself to the data and conservative interpretations. However, she sided with the brown bread lobby, believing that more vitamins could not help but be healthier. In her words, "The provision of National Wheatmeal bread by the authorities is a wise compromise, affording to a great extent the advantages of wholemeal bread in a form more acceptable to the general public."[17]

A Letter to the Editor

Harriette Chick could be moralistic. After her experience in Vienna after the First World War, she became concerned about food shortages in Europe during the Second. In November 1944, she, along with Charles Martin and Margaret Hume, wrote a letter to the editor of *The Times* expressing their concern.[18]

> It has been a surprise to many that, notwithstanding the tragic food shortage in many countries of Europe, the Food Minister should propose to increase, the rations for the British people at Christmas and that his proposals should have evoked relatively little public criticism.
>
> It is clear that many usually well informed people are not really alive to the state of affairs in Europe, or lack the spiritual vitality which would make them ashamed to receive an increase of their own

comparative plenty when others were looking starvation in the face. There can be no doubt of the facts. Although in certain agricultural districts there may be comparative plenty owing to the accumulations caused by breakdown of transport, the reports of severe food short-age have been confirmed by eye-witnesses who have recently visited large towns in Belgium, Holland, and Italy. The situation is known to be serious also in many districts of Greece and Yugoslavia and some districts of France. There is not only a shortage of special foods which could be met by more adequate distribution and by provision of special synthetic vitamins. The deficiency is of food, of any food and especially of bread and fats. Authentic stories are told of the children of even well-to-do families picking over the garbage bins near allied camps to relieve the pangs of hunger with any scraps of food they can find.

We have been and still are the best fed country of Europe, thanks to the efforts of the Royal and Merchant Navies, and to the enlightened policy of our Food Ministry which would be the first to acknowledge its debt to its scientific advisers and to the Government Committee on Scientific Food Policy. Thanks to these, we have been provided with an adequate ration of fats and a national bread of good quality which has remained unrationed. The same is true of our abundant potato supply, and no one need go hungry. Especially important foods such as milk, eggs, cheese, cod liver oil, and orange juice have been partially reserved for the priority classes that need them most.

Our population has not suffered in health from its war-time diet and one important class–the children–has improved in general health, stamina, growth, and development. Should we not, therefore, as a pro-fessedly Christian country continue to restrict ourselves to a diet that is adequate and healthy, and be willing to forgo any extra luxuries until our neighbours have enough plain food to nourish their bodies?
Yours very truly,
Charles J. Martin, Harriette Chick, E. Margaret Hume
Lister Institute of Preventive Medicine, Division of Nutrition, Roebuck House, Old Chesterton, Cambridge.

The letter, strong in Victorian moral values and weak in arguments likely to persuade a British public weary of wartime sacrifices, had no impact.

Post-War Bread

Everyone in Great Britain expected that things would get better after the war; and they did at first, if only marginally. The bread became a little paler and rose a bit better after the degree of extraction of the National Loaf was reduced first to 82.5% and then to 80%. This was done without publicity, but it caused a ruckus in Parliament when the brown bread advocates objected to the change. By many measures—infant and maternal mortality, the growth of children, the prevalence of anemia–the British population at the end of World War II was healthier than it had ever been.[19] Although many factors were responsible, some in Parliament attributed it to the adoption of the National Loaf and resisted any backsliding toward white bread. But the Ministry of Food persisted.

To prepare for peacetime, in January 1945 the Ministry of Food convened a conference to make recommendations for the post-war bread.[20] Harriette Chick was not invited; all the participants, except for the secretary, were men. Sir Edward Mellanby represented the MRC. In addition to government bureaucrats, representatives of millers, bakers, and grain and flour importers attended. No one represented the consumers, in particular the housewives responsible for food shopping and putting the meals on the table for their families.

The conferees assumed that the government would continue to regulate the bread supply, perhaps indefinitely. They recommended requiring bread to have the same nutritional value as the National Loaf, with prescribed minimum amounts of thiamin, nicotinic acid, and iron. These could be provided by flour of at least 80% extraction. The conference did not reach a firm conclusion as to whether white flour enriched with those nutrients would also be acceptable.

All of this became moot when wheat became even scarcer after the war than it had been during wartime. Having spent its money on the war, Great Britain was left with limited foreign exchange reserves to pay for imported grain. In addition to its own population, Great Britain was responsible for its colonies; and India was threatened with famine. European allies, devastated by the war, needed food. Even former enemies had to be fed, as each of the Allied powers assumed responsibility for a sector of a divided Germany. To make matters worse, the ravages of the war and a global drought resulted in a poor harvest in 1945 with a worldwide food shortage, especially of wheat.

As a result, food rationing in Great Britain did not end with victory.[21] A Labor government under Clement Attlee took office in July 1945, and not only continued food rationing, but made the rations skimpier than they had been in wartime. In May 1946, the wheat shortage forced the Ministry of Food to raise the extraction rate of flour to 90% and to reduce the weight of a standard loaf from 2 to 1.75 pounds, hoping that people would buy the same number of loaves. The consumption of bread actually increased, probably as a response to the reduction in other rationed foods.

In July 1946, the Ministry of Food instituted bread rationing. The primary motivation for this step is unclear. It may have been at least partially a dramatic gesture to persuade the United States to ship more wheat across the Atlantic. With better harvests, bread rationing ended in July 1948, but the Ministry of Food continued to require that only brown bread be sold. The extraction rate was decreased to 80% in 1950 and all restrictions were removed in 1956. The National Loaf became history and the country reverted to eating white bread.

After the war there was widespread belief that the National Loaf, despite its esthetic defects, had been important in keeping the civilian population healthy in the face of food shortages. Harriette Chick was given substantial credit for its adoption. In his 1949 Birthday Honors, the King awarded Harriette the title of Dame Commander (D.B.E.), a knighthood, "for services to the study of nutrition." She accepted the honor but disliked being addressed as Dame Harriette.

Coda

Harriette retired from the Lister Institute in 1945 at the age of seventy, five years after the standard retirement age. She moved to Cambridge, sharing a house with her widowed sister Elsie Blackman. However, she maintained an apartment in London and kept in contact with the Lister Institute. Although she no longer received a salary, she held the title of Honorary Member and retained her seat on the Council.

The Nutrition Division returned to London and, for a few years, continued to work on the nutritional value of proteins. Harriette maintained some contact with the laboratory and a few more papers were published with her listed as a co-author. The papers were of minor importance. The major developments in protein biology were being made at the molecular level, not in whole animals. The Nutrition Division atrophied and, after 1950, Harriette Chick and Margaret Hume were its only members and both were honorary.

Harriette remained an active member of the Nutrition Society, an organization she had helped to found. Membership had grown rapidly during the War, increasing from 179 original members to 600 in 1945. In recognition of her contributions, in 1949, she, along with Dr. Martin, was made an Honorary Member of the Society. Harriette went on to serve as its president from 1956 until 1959, when she was long retired from laboratory work and past her eightieth birthday.* Her major job as president was to organize meetings. Reflecting her interests, one session of a 1958 meeting was *Flour and Bread*. She led it off with a presentation titled "Wheat and bread. A historical introduction."[22]

She continued her interest in proteins and became particularly interested in the nutritive value of vegetable proteins for use in resource-limited environments where animal protein was too expensive. She studied a preparation of malted barley as a milk substitute.[23] One of her last papers, published in 1951, reviewed how to mix vegetable proteins to obtain a diet complete in essential amino acids.[24]

She had an opportunity to test her ideas. Between 1946 and 1948, she and Margaret Hume made several trips to Wuppertal, Germany, where the MRC had established a unit led by Elsie Widdowson and Robert A. McCance to study malnutrition, which was almost universal in post-war Germany.[25] As McCance and Widdowson wrote in the Preface to their report, they hoped to duplicate Harriette Chick's success in Vienna after World War I:

---

* The Nutrition Society denied me access to their archives, so this account relies on published sources.

Between 1919 and 1922 the Medical Research Council and the Lister Institute of Preventive Medicine maintained in Vienna a small team of British scientists engaged in the study of the deficiency diseases then prevalent in that part of Europe. The valuable results which Dame Harriette Chick and her colleagues achieved and the esteem in which they were held by the Viennese physicians among whom they worked, were a source of encouragement to the Council when, twenty years later it became necessary to prepare for similar work at the end of a second world war.[26]

The malnutrition in Wuppertal, however, was different from what Harriette Chick had encountered in Vienna. In Prof. von Piquet's Kinderklinik, the NEM system ensured that every child received sufficient calories and the Lister Institute investigators could study deficiencies of specific nutrients. Following World War II, there was not enough food of any kind in Germany. Children were unable to get sufficient calories or protein. This provided a different research opportunity than in post-World War I Vienna. In addition to studying the physiologic effects of protein-energy malnutrition, the Wuppertal investigators compared the ability of different diets to restore health.

In an effort to develop plant-based sources of protein, Harriette Chick and R. F. A. (Rex) Dean, one of the members of the Wuppertal team, designed experiments that tested mixtures of soya flour and malted cereals as a dietary supplement for malnourished children. There were limitations of the experiment, but the children did gain weight on the vegetable diets. Dean concluded, with some hedging, that: "It seems justifiable to conclude that if the mixture of amino acids is suitably adjusted, a diet entirely of plant origin can give excellent results, at least for short periods, in the feeding of children."[27] In Dean's later experience in Uganda, powdered milk proved a more practical source of protein.

The Wuppertal investigators also set out to confirm, in institutionalized children, Chick's finding that young rats grew better when fed wholemeal flour rather than white flour. The hope was to verify the superiority of brown bread in malnourished children by comparing different breads given to supplement the institutional diet in two orphanages.[28]

The children in the experiment, five to fifteen years of age, continued to receive the limited institutional rations, mainly vegetables, soup and potatoes, in amounts insufficient to support normal growth and development. At mealtimes, the children were divided into groups to compare different breads. Each group was assigned one kind of bread prepared from different flours, including wholemeal flour, 85% extraction brown flour, 70% extraction white flour, and white flour enriched with thiamin, niacin, nicotinic acid, riboflavin and iron. They were given as much bread as they wanted and, in addition, they all received supplements of calcium and vitamins A, D and C. For a year, the children's food consumption was charted daily and they were periodically weighed, measured, and their overall health assessed.

All the groups eagerly consumed the bread, which came to supply 75% of their total calories. All the children gained weight and improved in general health. However, the investigators were disappointed that there was no difference between the groups.

> *If one of the groups had made less progress than another it would in a way have made this a more satisfying experiment because, if it had shown conclusively the advantage of, let us say, wholemeal over white flour, the results of Chick's and other people's studies on growing rats would have been shown to apply to children. Experiments, however, are not made to give satisfaction but to win knowledge.*[29]

Being unable to demonstrate the superiority of wholemeal flour in children, they turned to rats to see if they could repeat Chick's findings. They first used 8-week-old rats and were unable to show a difference in the growth of those fed different flours. It was only when they duplicated Chick's experiment exactly, using 4-week-old rats immediately after weaning, that they could show the superiority of wholemeal flour. "Here then was a confirmation of Chick's findings, and a satisfactory demonstration (a) that there really were nutritional differences between the diets, (b) how very carefully the experimental setting had to be arranged in order to show them."[30]

Even McCance and Widdowson, who had been outspoken advocates of the National Loaf, accepted the results of the experiment in children. Harriette Chick's critics had been right. A small difference in the growth of weanling rats did not translate to humans eating a varied diet, even a diet deficient in calories and protein.

The Wuppertal investigators and the post-war food shortages brought protein malnutrition to the forefront of nutrition research. According to one researcher, the 1950s became the "protein decade."[31] The work in Wuppertal on plant proteins led R. F. A. Dean to move to Uganda, where *kwashiorkor*, a disease resulting from protein deficiency in post-weanling infants, was common. His efforts led to the establishment of the MRC Infantile Malnutrition Research Unit in Kampala.[32] This unit was to be instrumental in the understanding the physiology and treatment of kwashiorkor.

The Final Years

Harriette had an active retirement. She made periodic trips to Europe to visit friends and former colleagues. She was always happy to entertain friends and family in the house she shared with her sister in Cambridge. She was an avid gardener, and visitors for lunch or tea were first treated to a tour of her garden. Her other leisure activities were tennis and hiking. At some point she stopped attending church.[33] Apparently she did not retain the fundamentalist religious views of her father and Chick ancestors.

She never lost her interest in nutrition. In 1975, she was chosen to give the Prize Lecture to the British Nutrition Society. Two weeks before her hundredth birthday she introduced the lecture in person, although a colleague had to read it to the audience. It summarized her greatest success, her work in Vienna.[34]

Harriette Chick spent the last months of her life in a nursing home in Cambridge and died at a nephew's house in Uppercross, Cambridge, on July 9, 1977, at the age of 102. She was buried in a family plot in the churchyard of St. Mary's Perivale in Ealing, just north of the Notting Hill and Ealing High School. The tombstone, surrounded by stone crosses marking other graves, is notable for its lack of religious symbolism.

Her obituary in the *The Times* described her perfectly:

Dame Harriette was a person of quiet charm, of great determination, and of much courage. She had all the best and most sterling qualities of the Victorians – upright, honest, and, at all times, determined to do her duty.[35]

Notes

1   Hume, E. Margaret, and Chick, Harriette, eds., *Reports on Biological Standards IV.—The Standardization and Estimation of Vitamin A*. London: H. M. Stationery Office, 1935.

2   Copping AM (1978) The history of the Nutrition Society. *Proc Nutr Soc* 37: 105-139.

3   Anon. (1944) Meeting Report. *Proc Nutr Soc* 1 (1-2): 7-112

4   Chick H (1956) Charles James Martin 1866-1955. *Biographical Memoirs of Fellows of the Royal Society* 2: 173-208.

5   Copping AM (1990) Dame Harriette Chick. In: *The Nutrition Society. 1941-1991*, Elsie M. Widdowson, ed. (Oxford: CAB International, 1991), pp. 33-37.

6   Cooper S (1964)Snoek Piquante. In: Sissons, M., and French, P., eds., *The Age of Austerity* (Penguin Books: Middlesex, England), pp. 35-57.

7   Widdowson, E. M. (1936) A study of English diets by the individual method: Part I. Men. *J Hyg (Lond)* 36 (3): 269-292.

    Widdowson, E. M., and McCance, R. A. (1936) A study of the English diets by the individual method. Part II. Women. *J Hyg (Lond)* 36 (3): 293-309.

8   McCance R. A., and E. M. Widdowson (1956) *Breads White and Brown*. London: Pitman.

9   Chick, H. (1940) Nutritive value of white flour with vitamin B1 added and of whole-meal flour. *Lancet* 236 (6113): 511-512.

10 Wright MD (1941) The nutritive value of bread. Fortified white flour and national wheatmeal compared. *Br Med J* 2 (4219) 689-692.

    Chick H. (1941) The nutritive value of bread. *Br Med J* 2 (4221) 790-791.

11 Chick H (1942) Biological value of the proteins contained in wheat flours. *Lancet* 239 (6188): 405-407.

12 McCance RA, Widdowson EM (1942) Mineral metabolism of healthy adults on white and brown bread dietaries. *J Physiol* 101: 44-85.

13 Medical Research Council (1940) Improved quality of bread. Higher extraction of flour. *Br Med J* 2 (4152): 164.

    Medical Research Council (1941) National Flour for bread. MRC specifications. *Br Med J* 1 (4195): 828-829.

14 Medical Research Council (1941) National Flour for bread. MRC specifications. *Br Med J* 1 (4195): 828-829.

    Medical Research Council (1941) National flour. A second memorandum. *Lancet* 237 (6144): 703-704

15 Anon. (1942) *Brit Food J* 44 (4) 31-40.

16 The wheatmeal loaf. *The Manchester Guardian*, March 23, 1942.

17   Chick H (1942) Biological value of the proteins contained in wheat flours. *Lancet*
     239 (6188): 405-407.

18   Martin CJ, Chick H, Hume EM (1944) The British rations. Letter to the Editor. *The
     Times of London*, November 14, 1944.

19   Sitwell, William (1988) *Eggs or Anarchy* (New York: Simon and Schuster), pp.
     228-229.

20   Ministry of Food (1945) *Report of the Conference on the Post-War Loaf.* Cmd. 6701.
     London: H. M. Stationery Office.

21   Cooper S. (1963) Snoek Piquante. In: Sissons, M., and French. P. (eds.) *Age of
     Austerity. 1945-1951*, Middlesex, England: Penguin Books.

22   Chick H (1958) Wheat and bread. A historical introduction. *Proc Nutr Soc* 17 (1): 1-7.

23   Chick H, Slack EB (1946) Malted foods for Babies. Trials with young rats. *Lancet*
     248 (6426): 601-603.

24   Chick, H (1951) Nutritive value of vegetable proteins and its enhancement by admix-
     ture. *Br J Nutr* 5(2): 261-265.

25   Widdowson EM (1992) Undernutrition in Germany in the post-war period. In: E.

     M. Widdowson and J. Mathers, eds., *The Contributions of Nutrition to Human and
     Animal health* (Cambridge: Cambridge University Press), pp. 293-302.

26   Medical Research Council (1951) *Studies of Undernutrition, Wuppertal 1946-9.*
     Medical Research Council Special Reports Series No. 275 (London: His Majesty's
     Stationery Office), p. v-vi.

27   Dean RFA (1951) The nutritional adequacy of a vegetable substitute for milk. *Br J
     Nutrition* 5 (2): 269-274.

28   McCance, R. A., and Widdowson, E. M. (1956) *Breads White and Brown. Their
     Place in Thought and Social History* (London: Pitman Medical Publishing Co. Ltd.),
     pp. 120-123.

29   McCance, R. A., and Widdowson, E. M. (1956) *Breads White and Brown*, p. 123.

30   McCance, R. A., and Widdowson, E. M. (1956) *Breads White and Brown*, p. 125.

31   Brock JF (1961) Dietary proteins in relation to man's health. *Fed Proc* 20 (1): 61-65.

32   Widdowson EM (1991) Dame Harriette Chick. In: *The Nutrition Society 1941-1991.*
     Elsie M. Widdowson, ed. (Oxford: C.A.B. International, 1991), p. 37.

33   Chick, Jonathan, personal communication, 3 March 2020.

34   Chick H (1976) Study of rickets in Vienna 1919-1922. *Med Hist* 20: 41-51.

35   *The Times of London*, July 11, 1977.

CHAPTER 11
LEGACY

Breaking Barriers

The term scientist did not exist until it was coined in 1834 by the English philosopher William Whewell.[1] Those who studied the natural world called themselves *natural philosophers* or *men of science*. Indeed, almost all were men and most were wealthy. Not needing to earn a living, they conducted research at their own expense, purely for the love of discovery. The term scientist was readily accepted in the United States, but many in Britain resisted using the new word, either because they did not like the way it sounded or because it implied that they were motivated by money.

During the second half of the nineteenth century, some men began to earn a living doing science. Universities, monarchs, government agencies, the military and industry began to pay them to do research in support of their varied missions. Over time, the wealthy amateurs stopped looking down on the professionals.

Throughout the eighteenth and nineteenth centuries, women also followed in the tradition of unpaid science. Among the upper classes, a proper woman did not stoop to doing remunerative work. Wealthy women, such as the mathematician Ada Lovelace (Ada King, Countess of Lovelace), paid for their research out of their own, or their husbands', pockets. The less fortunate, such as the paleontologist Mary Anning, made do with scarce resources. She raised money by selling the dinosaur bones she discovered to museums and collectors.

The result was that, until the twentieth century, few women were paid to do science. Marie Curie (1867-1934), who worked in France, was the best known; and there were a handful in the United States, most notably the archeologist Erminnie A. Smith (1836-1886) at the Smithsonian Institution. The lone exception in Great Britain was Caroline Herschel, the sister of the astronomer William Herschel. In 1787. King George III awarded her an annual salary of £50 to assist her brother. By the turn of the twentieth century, a handful of British women held university faculty appointments; but they had heavy teaching loads and could do little research.

As best as I can ascertain, Harriette Chick was the first female professional scientist in Great Britain since Caroline Herschel. Harriette not only achieved her ambition of becoming a scientist, but she also became head of a laboratory and director of a division of a major research institution She was the first woman in Great Britain to achieve this status. Her work made a major impact on medical science and public health. Her success paved the way for other women.

At the Lister Institute, once the men on the staff discovered that they could work alongside a woman, others were hired without opposition. In 1909, Muriel Robertson (1883-1973), a protozoologist, came on board, first as an assistant and promoted to the staff a year later. Supported by the Royal Society, she went to Uganda from 1911 to 1913, where she did seminal work on trypanosomiasis (African sleeping sickness). In contrast to Harriette Chick's modesty, Muriel Robertson was brash and outspoken. According to Harriette, her "zest was to add spice to the institute for many years."[2]

Following World War I, they were the only two women on the permanent staff of the Lister Institute; but at least it was a beginning. Harriette's assistants in her laboratory were almost all women, probably because men were willing to work alongside women but unwilling to be bossed by one. Nevertheless, the men soon realized that women's minds were as suited for rigorous scientific thought as their own. Britain could not afford to allow such a pool of talent to lie idle, especially during wartime. More and more women took up careers as investigators. Even now women in science face more obstacles than men and their numbers remain fewer; but they now have a pathway to a successful career thanks to Harriette Chick and her fellow pioneers.[3]

Why Harriette Chick

What allowed Harriette to break through when others ran up against the wall of sexism? Four factors had to combine to allow Harriette Chick to blaze the trail: intelligence, focus, courage, and luck.

First, she had intelligence and self-discipline. She was a star student from primary school through university, but she was not a genius. She did not spark new ways of thinking about nutrition. The basic ideas about vitamins had been expounded before she entered the field. Her meticulous experiments confirmed those ideas at a time when there was widespread skepticism, but she did not break new ground.

In addition to being smart, she remained focused. She fell in love with science at the Notting Hill High School and single-mindedly pursued a career in biology. When Bedford College did not live up to her expectations, she relinquished a scholarship to transfer to UCL, where science and math were much stronger. Importantly, she never married and devoted her energy to her career.

However, there were many equally intelligent British women of her era. Others who aspired to be scientists fell by the wayside, while Harriette went on to a distinguished career. Two other factors set her apart: her courage and her extraordinary good luck.

She demonstrated courage in large and small ways. Taking the job at the Lister Institute in the face of opposition from some of the faculty required bravery. One of her first publications after joining the Lister Institute was a study in which Harriette offered her forearm to be bitten by fleas as part of Martin's investigation of an epidemic of plague in India. When she put her arm in a cage of fleas, "many...could be felt at once to bite vigorously." [4]

She also showed courage in large ways, particularly in her travels. In 1918, against Dr. Martin's advice, she left a comfortable life in London to go to war-torn Vienna. Eastern Europe after World War I was impoverished and dangerous. Governments could not maintain order and robbery was common. But Harriette saw an opportunity to contribute to science and to public health and accepted the risks.

Her courage allowed her to take advantage of the remarkable luck she enjoyed throughout her life. She had the good fortune to be born into an unusual family for their times. The Chicks had a heritage of strong women and expected them to be leaders. Furthermore, Samuel and Emma could afford to send their daughters to expensive schools to develop their leadership skills. Samuel's fortuitous encounter with Lady Stanley proved a key event, resulting in the enrollment of his daughters in the Notting Hill High School, which dared to teach math and science to girls.

Perhaps Harriette's greatest stroke of luck was working in a laboratory downstairs from the giant of neurophysiology, Charles Sherrington, whom she befriended and impressed with her intelligence and diligence. Sherrington's letter of recommendation earned her a position at the Lister Institute. Harriette Chick had the knack for being in the right place at the right time.

This knack also bore fruit when she ventured to Vienna after World War I. The widespread malnutrition, the unique facility she encountered at the Kinderklinik, and the support she received from Prof. von Piquet and the Viennese medical community could not have been duplicated anywhere else. She left London with only a vague idea of what she would find, but she went with a prepared mind and made the most of her good fortune.

Her Science

The epigraph for this book is a quotation from a paper by the historian of science Thomas Haskins. He makes two points: first, the careers of scientists frequently take unexpected turns; and, second, science is heavily influenced by the events and values of the society in which the scientist is immersed. Harriette Chick's career illustrates both conclusions.

It was natural that Harriette was first attracted to bacteriology. At the end of the nineteenth century, the germ theory was the dominant paradigm of medical science and microorganisms were thought to explain virtually every human disease. Ambitious students who wanted to be on the cutting edge of medical science aspired to discover the germs that caused the illnesses that remained mysterious.

Harriette's first attempts as a graduate student, focused on polluted water and its purification, were rigorous but judged to be unimportant. They taught her how to design and conduct experiments but did not lead to a sustainable line of research. It was only when she joined the Lister Institute that she blossomed into a productive independent investigator.

When biochemistry was in its infancy, her studies of disinfection and protein denaturation, done in collaboration with Charles Martin, were crucial in understanding these processes. Their papers were among the first to apply quantitative analysis to biological problems, at the time a revolutionary concept. These early papers led to her being inducted into the Biochemical Society and could have easily led to a productive career in basic biochemistry. However, World War I intervened and her career pivoted unexpectedly.

Harriette welcomed the move to nutrition research and it turned out to be another stroke of luck, allowing her to not only be at the forefront of another branch of medical science but to be the head of a major research program. Again, Charles Martin was her benefactor. It was because he was assigned to the Australian military hospital on Lemnos and because the work of Funk and Cooper at the Lister Institute had taught him about beriberi that he told Harriette to stop manufacturing antisera and get back to doing original science. She made the most of her opportunity.

Although clinical nutrition research now occupies a minor position in biological science, at the turn of the last century the study of vitamins was exciting science. In the major biochemistry and physiology journals, nutrition studies filled a large portion of their pages. That a person could enjoy a diet with abundant calories and still suffer malnutrition was revolutionary at a time when microorganisms were invoked to explain every human malady. Scurvy, beriberi, and pellagra were all blamed on infections. The recognition of vitamin deficiency diseases and the isolation and chemical characterization of vitamins was an important chapter, now little appreciated, in the history of medical science.

Due to Charles Martin's mandate to lead nutrition research at the Lister Institute, Harriette Chick caught the crest of the wave of interest in vitamins. She carried out her research when many vitamin deficiency diseases were still common. Rickets, hunger osteomalacia, and pellagra were prevalent in Europe and North America; and infantile scurvy and vitamin A deficiency occurred in times of famine.

In Vienna, she had an ample supply of subjects for clinical trials. She also had the advantage of conducting her clinical trials in institutionalized populations. We no longer have orphanages and ethical standards for conducting research in institutionalized populations have evolved, so that type of research is no longer feasible.

Harriette Chick could put her work into context, but she was justifiably proud of her accomplishments. She wrote:

Perhaps the greatest contribution of the Lister team's work on rickets was to the public health. Many others contributed to the complete picture of scientific fact, particularly Edward Mellanby in England and scientists and paediatricians in the United States. The Vienna experiments were unique in providing a dramatic and easily comprehensible demonstration that rickets can be prevented or cured equally by cod-liver oil or by ultra-violet light. It was no longer necessary for stunted and bowlegged men and women to be seen every day in the streets.[5]

The crest of the wave of interest in vitamins passed and Harriette achieved little of major scientific importance after she returned from Vienna; but for over a decade she was at exactly the right intellectual place at the right time, contributing to a revolution in medical science and the almost complete elimination of vitamin deficiency diseases from the developed world.

These diseases had killed and disabled millions over the eighteenth and nineteenth centuries. Only vaccination and modern sanitation have had bigger impacts on public health. However, her very success led to her name fading from accounts of the history of medicine. As vitamin deficiency diseases disappeared from public view, the names of early twentieth century investigators who conquered those diseases also disappeared from textbooks and lectures.

The Men in Her Life

The most important man in Harriette's adult life was Charles James Martin. Margaret Hume, in her obituary of Martin, wrote:

I first met Professor Martin in 1911 when, with Harriette Chick and her young sister, I attended a meeting of the British Association at

Portsmouth. I was deeply impressed when Harriette Chick gave a paper
on the work she had been doing with Martin on the mechanism and
rate of the coagulation of proteins by heat (Chick & Martin, 1912).[6]
She held the position of Assistant to the Director, and continued to do
so officially until he retired in January 1931, and unofficially as long as
he lived.[7]

Charles Martin deserves substantial credit for Harriette's success. He
hired her over the objections of some of his colleagues and mentored her
throughout their time together at the Lister Institute and after, when the
Nutrition Department relocated to his estate in Cambridge during World
War II. Harriette made no important professional decisions without consult-
ing the Boss. Even though she did not always follow his advice, she continued
to value his counsel and remained a close friend until he died in 1955. When
separated geographically, notably during wartime, they maintained an active
correspondence. However, there is no evidence that their relationship was
other than platonic.

Except during World War I, the number of women on the professional
staff of the Lister Institute never exceeded a small minority. But Charles
Martin at least opened the door. As Director of the pre-eminent medical
research institute in Great Britain, he appointed first Harriette and then other
women to the staff. Muriel Robertson joined the staff in 1909, shortly after
Harriette Chick's promotion, and later became the head of the Department of
Protozoology. Others were to follow in bacteriology and biochemistry. There
are few clues in Martin's biography as to what made him open-minded when
sexism dominated English professional life.

Charles Martin was not the only man with whom Harriette formed a
close professional relationship and who proved instrumental in her career.
Charles Sherrington was key at the beginning of her career and Clemens von
Pirquet during her work on rickets in Vienna. Her ability to work produc-
tively in collaboration with male colleagues was no doubt essential in opening
the door for more women in science.

Honors

Although few current scientists or physicians have heard of Harriette Chick, at the time her work was valued by her colleagues. After she retired, she was a respected emerita of the Lister Institute, retaining a title as Honorary Member and a seat on the Council. She received Royal honors, first C.B.E. and then D.B.E. She was elected to the Biochemical Society and was a founding member of the Nutrition Society. The Nutrition Society made her an Honorary Member after she retired from the Lister Institute and she later served as its president.

However, despite her impact on medical science and public health, she did not receive the Nobel Prize, while others less deserving, such as F. Gowland Hopkins, did. Kenneth Carpenter, an expert on the history of vitamins, in his essay about Nobel Prizes for nutrition research, wrote of the deliberations of the Nobel Prize Committee:

> Among the important advances made in this field between the time of Hopkins' work and the 1929 awards was the work on the fat-soluble vitamins begun by McCollum and followed up by many others. For example, Harriette Chick had led a team, during the post-World War I food crisis in Central Europe, who studied the treatment of rickets in Vienna and showed, using X-rays, that bone healing in infants was equally stimulated by ultraviolet irradiation or dosing with cod liver oil, and had nothing to do with hygiene. Nevertheless, the Committee in the following years decided, it seems, that this period of work on vitamins had now been adequately recognized. [8]

Carpenter goes on to comment on the award of the 1934 Prize to George Whipple, George Minot, and William Murphy, who cured pernicious anemia by feeding patients liver extract. Their discovery was no more fundamental than Harriette Chick's prevention of rickets with cod liver oil; but the cure of pernicious anemia, a fatal illness when untreated, was far more dramatic than the prevention of a chronic disease that only affected the bones. And whereas Harriette Chick's work was not paradigm-shifting, Whipple, Minot and Murphy demonstrated that a disease that many thought was malignant could be treated with dietary manipulation. They produced a dramatic shift in the view of a common, fatal disease and, therefore, were deemed more deserving of recognition than Harriette.

Values and Personal Life

Harriette Chick was a product of the Victorian era. In keeping with her time and station, she had a strong sense of duty. When called upon, she sacrificed for the common good. She gave up her productive biochemical studies to do routine work manufacturing antisera when World War I broke out. Then, when Charles Martin asked, she pivoted again to nutrition research to help feed the soldiers. When the war ended and the MRC called on her to go to Vienna, she again accepted the challenge despite the personal risk. Once in Vienna, affected by widespread deprivation, she tried doing some unofficial relief work with children in addition to her scientific studies. She only gave those efforts up when she felt betrayed by people back in England. And during World War II, she turned her laboratory efforts to studying how to nourish a civilian population faced with a shortage of food.

She consistently devoted her scientific efforts to addressing pressing problems of public health, whether it was polluted water, killing infectious microbes, or malnutrition. Even in retirement, when she could have just tended her garden in Cambridge, she did her duty by taking on the presidency of the Nutrition Society, an organization she had helped to found.

She was also Victorian in her dress and manners. According to her relative, Dr. Jonathan Chick, who visited her during her retirement in Cambridge, her dress was "from another generation."[9] The surviving photographs show her in long skirts and high-collared blouses, typically looking down at a book or at her work. She was as modest in her manner as in her dress. She wrote little, even in her diaries, about her personal life. In retirement she resisted being addressed as Dame Harriette. This modesty likely contributed to her acceptance in a predominantly male culture. She worked diligently in her laboratory, and, except for Charles Martin, almost exclusively with other women. She did not threaten the men working on their own projects.

However, her modesty contributed to my greatest disappointment researching this book: I could learn little of Harriette Chick's inner life. Harriette's niece Margaret Tomlinson, who wrote the Chick family history, suffered the same disappointment. She lamented the scarcity of family papers and letters. As she said, the Chicks were hardworking, practical people who did not write about themselves.

> *Even if they had kept intimate diaries or written long revealing letters to one another—which is doubtful—such evidence would afterwards have been scrupulously destroyed. Moreover the Chick women, like good housewives, were always clearing out and throwing away. The few documents which have escaped seem to have done so almost by accident.[10]*

Did Harriette Chick ever have a romantic relationship? None are mentioned in her surviving diaries, nor are any noted in her obituaries. If she had a trove of letters from admirers, they have disappeared. Her life revolved around work and family. Her unmarried state gave her opportunities in a society in which married women were excluded from the professions; but it is unclear if this was a deliberate choice or a lack of opportunity. The conflict between demanding careers, including those in science, and family responsibilities continues to be a special problem for women.[11] Harriette avoided the conflict by never marrying.

Another gap in the record is the role of religion in her adult life. She was raised in a strict Baptist household, with frequent prayers and church attendance. Worldly entertainment was forbidden. She made notes of attending church in her Vienna diaries. Furthermore, these diaries contain curious markings in the corners of some pages, including are crosses with other associated peculiar marks that appear religious in nature. However, she stopped attending church by the time she retired to Cambridge. She was buried in the family plot in a churchyard of an Anglican parish, along with her father, mother and siblings. Apparently, Samuel, a staunch Baptist and one-time member of the Passive Resistance League, mellowed in his opposition to the Church of England in his old age. It is unlikely that his family would have buried him in an Anglican churchyard against his wishes.

Harriette's life revolved around family and work. As was typical for an unmarried woman of her time and social class, she lived with her parents and unmarried sisters when she was not traveling. Her work revolved around the Lister Institute, to which she was devoted. She was quite proud of her accomplishments and there is little doubt that she entered retirement quite content with the choices she had made.

Courage and Luck

Harriette Chick's story, like that of many pioneers, is a story of courage and determination. It illustrates the challenges faced by an ambitious Englishwoman at the beginning of the twentieth century and the extraordinary conjunction of circumstances that had to combine to allow a woman born in Great Britain in 1875, even a woman with Harriette Chick's exceptional qualities, to achieve professional success.

One can only lament the waste of talent that resulted from excluding half of the population from careers in science. It is also lamentable that it required two world wars to change the status quo. Women scientists continue to face more obstacles than their male counterparts, but they now achieve positions of leadership and their contributions are recognized with prestigious appointments and prizes. It is thanks to Harriette Chick and the other women brave enough, determined enough, and talented enough to enter the first wave of women in science that the barriers began to be eroded.

Notes

1   Ross S (1962) *Scientist:* the story of a word. *Ann Science* 18 (2): 65-85.

2   Chick, Harriette, Margaret Hume and Marjorie Macfarlane (1971) *War on Disease. A History of the Lister Institute* (London: Andre Deutch), p. 75.

3   Graham PA (1970) Women in academe. *Science* 169 (3952): 1284-1290.

4   Chick H, Martin CJ (1911) The fleas common on rats in different parts of the world and the readiness with which they bite man. *J Hyg (Lond)* 11 (1): 122-136.

5   Chick H et al. (1971) *War on Disease*, p. 160.

6   Chick H, Martin CJ (1912) On the "heat coagulation" of proteins. Part IV. The conditions controlling the agglutination of proteins already acted upon by hot water. *J Physiol* 45 (4): 261-295.

7   Hume EM (1956) Obituary. Charles James Martin, Kt, C.M.G, F.R.C.P, D.Sc., F.R.S. (9 January 1866-15 February 1955) *Br J Nutr* 10 (1): 1-7.

8   Carpenter KJ (2004) The Nobel Prize and the discovery of vitamins. <https://www.nobelprize.org/prizes/themes/the-nobel-prize-and-and-the-discovery-of-vitamins>

9   Chick, Jonathan, personal communication, 3 March 2020.

10   Tomlinson, Margaret (1985) *Three Generations in the Honiton Lace Trade* (Sidmouth: Sovereign Printing Group), p. 1.

11   Goldin, Claudia (2021) *Career & Family. Women's Century-Long Journey toward Equity.* Princeton: Princeton University Press.

ACKNOWLEDGEMENTS

This biography relies primarily on published sources. Aside from Harriette Chick's scientific papers, the most important were *Three Generations in the Honiton Lace Trade*, the Chick family history written by Harriette's niece, Margaret Tomlinson, and *War on Disease. A History of the Lister Institute*, written by Harriette and her long-time colleagues Margaret Hume and Majorie Macfarlane. In tracking down more obscure references, I am grateful for the help of librarians at the University of California, Berkeley, Biosciences, Natural Resources and Public Health Library and the Harvard University Countway Library of Medicine.

The most important trove of unpublished materials pertaining to Harriette Chick is housed at the incomparable Wellcome Collection in London. It has some of Harriette's Chick's materials from the Lister Institute and has preserved the notebook of her trip to Germany in 1906 as well as her personal diaries from years 1916-1922, spanning her time in Vienna. In addition to its vast library, the Wellcome Collection provides a staff of professional librarians and unmatched facilities for researchers to explore its holdings. I also benefitted from the records of the 1851 Exhibition Commission, cheerfully aided by their archivist Angela Kenney, and from holdings of the National Archives of Great Britain.

Jonathan Chick and Gillian Lumb, relatives of Harriette Chick who knew her in life, were generous in sharing personal reminiscences. Barbara

Farquharson of the Branscombe Project sent me copies of photographs of Harriette and letters to her sister Edith found in trunks recovered from an attic in Margaret Tomlinson's house in Branscombe.

Cristen Iris, editor extraordinaire, helped make the story of Harriette Chick's life and science more coherent than my early efforts. My writers' group—Michael Larsen, Richard Bailey, Keh-Ming Lin, Jane Pearson, and Sydney Sauber—provided many helpful editorial suggestions. Kiran Spees of Fukurou Design Studio made the book look good. Troy Lamber and Stacey Smekofske (Edits by Stacey) performed copy editing and proof reading. I took most of their excellent suggestions, but stubbornly resisted some. Do not blame them when the text does not adhere to any accepted style manual.

Peter Reed, a friend, a professional historian of science, and a native Brit, provided a sounding board and helped me navigate institutions, literature, and the London Underground.

Most of all, I thank my wife, Susan Semonoff, who never complained about the time and money spent on this project.

BIBLIOGRAPHY

Harriette Chick's Publications

Chick H (1900) The distribution of Bacterium coli commune. *The Thompson-Yates Laboratories Report* 3 (1):1-29.

Chick, H (1902-03) A study of unicellular green alga, occurring in polluted water, with especial reference to its nitrogen metabolism. *Proc Roy Soc London* 71: 458-476.

Chick H (1905) The biological limitations of the method of pure culture. *The New Phytologist* 4 (5/6): 120-124.

Chick H (1906) A study of the process of nitrification with reference to the purification of sewage. *Proc Roy Soc London Series B* 77(517): 241-266.

Chick H (1908) An investigation of the laws of disinfection. *J Hyg (Lond)* 8 (1): 92-158.

Chick H, Martin CJ (1908a) The principles involved in the standardization of disinfectants and the influence of organic matter upon germicidal value. *J Hyg (Lond)* 8 (5): 654-697.

Chick H, Martin CJ (1908b) A comparison of the power of a germicide emulsified or dissolved, with an interpretation of the superiority of the emulsified form. *J Hyg (Lond)* 8 (5): 698-703.

Chick H (1910) The process of disinfection by chemical agencies and hot water. *J Hyg (Lond)* 10 (2): 237-286.

Chick H, Martin CJ (1910) On the "heat coagulation" of proteins. *J Physiol* 40 (5): 404-430.

Chick H, Martin CJ (1911) On the "heat-coagulation of proteins: Part II. The action of hot water upon egg-albumin and the influence of acid and salts upon reaction velocity. *J Physiol* 43 (1): 1-27.

Chick H, Martin CJ (1911) The fleas common in rats in different parts of the world and the readiness with which they bite man. *J Hyg (Lond)* 11 (1): 122-136.

Chick H (1912) The bactericidal properties of blood serum. I. The reaction-velocity of the germicidal action of normal rabbit serum on *B. coli commune* and the influence of temperature thereon. *J Hyg (Lond)* 12 (4): 414-435.

Chick H, Martin CJ (1912a) On the "heat-coagulation" of proteins: Part III. The influence of alkali upon reaction velocity. *J Physiol* 45 (1-2): 61-69.

Chick H, Martin CJ (1912b) On the "heat coagulation" of proteins: Part IV. The conditions controlling the aggregation of proteins already acted upon by hot water. *J Physiol* 45 (4): 261-295.

Chick H (1913) The factors concerned in the solution and precipitation of euglobulin. *Biochem J* 7 (3): 318-340.

Chick H, Martin CJ (1913a) The density and solution volume of some proteins. *Biochem J* 7 (1): 92-96.

Chick H, Martin CJ (1913b) The precipitation of egg-albumin by ammonium sulphate. A contribution to the theory of the "salting-out" of proteins. *Biochem J* 7 (4): 380-398.

Chick H, Martin CJ (1913c) *Die Hitzekoagulation der Eiweisskörper.* Dresden: Theodor Steinkopf.

Chick H (1914a) The viscosity of protein solutions. II. Pseudoglobulin and euglobulin (horse). *Biochem J* 8 (3): 261-280.

Chick H (1914b) The apparent formation of euglobulin from pseudo-globulin and a suggestion as to the relationship between these two proteins in serum. *Biochem J* 8 (4): 404-420.

Chick H, Lubrzynska E (1914) The viscosity of some protein solutions. *Biochem J* 8 (1): 59-69.

Chick H (1916) The preparation and use of certain agglutinating sera. *Lancet* 187 (4834): 857-861.

Chick H, Hume M (1917) The distribution among foodstuffs (especially those suitable for the rationing of armies) of the substances required for the prevention of (a) beriberi and (b) scurvy. *Trans Soc Trop Med Hyg* 10 (8): 141-186; *Journal of the Royal Army Medical Corps* 29 (2): 121-159.

Chick H, Hume M (1917) The distribution in wheat, rice, and maize grains of the substance, the deficiency of which in a diet causes polyneuritis in birds and beri-beri in man. *Proc Royal Society London* 90: 44-60.

Chick H, Hume M (1917) The effect of exposure to temperatures at or above 100° C. upon the substance (vitamine) whose deficiency in a diet causes polyneuritis in birds and beri-beri in man. *Proc Royl Soc London Series B* 90: 60-68.

Chick H, Hume EM, Skelton RF (1918) The anti-scorbutic value of cow's milk. *Biochem J* 12 (1-2): 131-153.

Chick H, Hume EM, Slelton RF (1918) An estimate of the antiscorbutic value of milk in infant feeding. *Lancet* 191 (4923): 1-2.

Chick H, Hume EM, Skelton RF, Henderson Smith A (1918) The relative content of antiscorbutic principle in limes and lemons, together with some new facts and some old observations concerning the value of "lime juice" in the prevention of scurvy. *Lancet* 192 (4970): 735-738.

Chick H, Rhodes M. (1918) An investigation of the antiscorbutic value of the raw juices of root vegetables, with a view to their adoption as an adjunct to the dietary of infants. *Lancet* 192 (4971): 774-775.

Campbell MED, Chick H (1919) I. The antiscorbutic and growth-promoting value of canned vegetables. *Lancet* 194 (5008): 320-322.

Chick H, Hume EM, Skelton RF (1919) II. The antiscorbutic value of some

Indian dried fruits: (a) tamarind, (b) cocum, and (c) mango ("amchur"). *Lancet* 194 (5008): 322-323.

Chick H, Delf EM (1919) The anti-scorbutic value of dry and germinated seeds. *Biochem J* 13 (2): 199-218.

Chick H, Hume EM (1919) Note on the importance of accurate and quantitative measurements in experimental work on nutrition and accessory food factors. *J Biol Chem* 39 (2): 203-207.

Chick H, Dalyell EJ (1920) The influence of overcooking vegetables in causing scurvy among children. *Br Med J* 2 (3119): 546-548.

Chick H, Hume EM (1920) The production in monkeys of symptoms closely resembling those of pellagra, by prolonged feeding on a diet of low protein content. *Biochem J* 14 (2): 135-146.

Dalyell EJ, Chick H (1921) Hunger-osteomalacia in Vienna, 1920.: 1.—Its relation to diet. *Lancet* 198 (5121): 842-849.

Chick H, Dalyell EJ (1921) Observations on the influence of foods rich in accessory food factors in stimulating development in backward children. *Br Med J* 2 (3182): 1061-1066.

Chick M, Dalyell EJ, Hume M, Mackay HMM, Henderson Smith H, Wimberger H. (1922) The etiology of rickets in infants: prophylactic and curative observations at the Vienna University Kinderklinik. *Lancet* 200 (5157): 7-11.

Chick H et al. (1923) *Studies of rickets in Vienna 1919-1922: report to the Accessory Food Factors Committee appointed jointly by the Medical Research Council and the Lister Institute.* London: H.M. Stationery Office.

Chick H (1924) Discussion on nutritional diseases in animals. *Proc Roy Soc Med* 17 (Sect Comp Med): 25-27.

Boas MA, Chick H (1924) The influence of diet and management of the cow upon the deposition of calcium in rats receiving a daily ration of the milk in their diet. *Biochem J* 18 (2): 433-447.

Chick H (1926) Sources of error in the technique employed for the biological assay of fat-soluble vitamins. *Biochem J* 20 (1): 119-130.

Chick H, Korenchevsky V, Roscoe MH (1926) The difference in chemical composition of the skeletons of young rats fed (1) on diets deprived of fat-soluble vitamins and (2) on a low phosphorus rachitic diet, compared with those of normally nourished animals of the same age. *Biochem J* 20 (3): 622-631.

Chick H, Roscoe MH (1926a) The anti-rachitic value of fresh spinach. *Biochem J* 20 (1): 137-152.

Chick H, Roscoe MH (1926b) Influence of diet and sunlight upon the amount of vitamin A and vitamin D in the milk afforded by a cow. *Biochem J* 20 (3): 632-649.

Henderson Smith H, Chick H (1926) Maintenance of a standardized breed of young rats for work upon fat-soluble vitamins, with particular reference to the endowment of the offspring. *Biochem J* 20 (1) 131-136.

Chick H (1927) The bactericidal properties of blood serum. I. The reaction-velocity of the germicidal action of normal rabbit-serum on *B. coli commune* and the influence of temperature thereon. *J Hyg (Lond)* 12 (4): 414-435.

Chick H, Roscoe MH (1927) On the composite nature of the water-soluble B vitamin. *Biochem J* 21 (3): 698-711.

Chick H, Roscoe MH (1928) The dual nature of water-soluble vitamin B. II: The effect upon young rats of vitamin B(2) deficiency and a method for the biological assay of vitamin B(2). *Biochem J* 22 (3): 790-799.

Chick H (1929) Clemens Pirquet and his work: director of the Vienna University Kinder-Klinik, 1911-1929. *Lancet* 213 (5508): 624-626.

Chick H (1929) The effect on vitamin B(2) of treatment with nitrous acid. *Biochem J* 23 (3): 514-516.

Chick H, Roscoe MH (1929a) A method for the assay of the anti-neuritic vitamin B(1), in which the growth of young rats is used as a criterion. *Biochem J* 23 (3): 498-503.

Chick H, Roscoe MH (1929b) An attempt to separate vitamin B(2) from vitamin B(1) in yeast and a comparison of its properties with those of the antineuritic vitamin B(1). *Biochem J* 23 (3): 504-513.

Chick H, Copping AM (1930a) The heat-stability of the (anti-dermatitis, "anti-pellagra") water-soluble vitamin B(2). I. *Biochem J* 24 (1): 105-112.

Chick H, Copping AM (1930b) The heat-stability of the (anti-dermatitis, "anti-pellagra") water-soluble vitamin B(2). II. *Biochem J* 24 (4): 932-938.

Chick H, Copping AM (1930c) The alcohol-stability of the anti-dermatitis, more heat-stable vitamin B(2) constituent of the vitamin B complex. *Biochem J* 24 (6): 1744-1747.

Chick H, Copping AM (1930d) The composite nature of the water-soluble vitamin B: Dietary factors in addition to the anti-neuritic vitamin B(1) and the anti-dermatitis vitamin B(2). *Biochem J* 24 (6): 1764-1769.

Chick H, Copping AM, Roscoe MH (1930) Egg-white as a source of the anti-dermatitis vitamin B(2). *Biochem J* 24 (6): 1748-1753.

Chick H, Roscoe MH (1930a) The heat-stability of the (anti-dermatitis, "anti-pellagra") water-soluble vitamin B(2). *Biochem J* 24: 105-112.

Chick H, Roscoe MH (1930b) The biological value of proteins: a method for measuring the nitrogenous exchange rate of rats for the purpose of determining the biological value of proteins. *Biochem J* 24 (6): 1780-1782.

Chick H (1932) The relation of ultra-violet light to nutrition. *Lancet* 220 (5685): 325-330.

Chick H, Jackson HM (1932) Note on the international standard for the anti-neuritic vitamin B(1). *Biochem J* 26 (4): 1223-1226.

Chick H (1933) Current theories of pellagra. *Lancet* 222 (5737): 341-346.

Chick H (1935) Diet and climate. *Current Science* 4 (5): 343-344.

Chick H, Boas-Fixsen MA, Hutchinson JCD, Jackson HM (1935) The biological value of proteins: the influence of variation in the level of protein in the diet and of heating the protein on its biological value. *Biochem J* 29 (7): 1712-1919.

Chick H, Copping AM, Edgar CE (1935) The water-soluble B vitamins. IV. The components of vitamin B(2). *Biochem J* 29 (3): 722-734.

Chick H, Hutchinson JCD, Jackson HM (1935) The biological value of proteins:

VI. further investigation of the balance sheet method. *Biochem J* 29 (7): 1702-1711.

Chick H (1937) The aetiology of pellagra. *Lancet* 229 (5928) 900.

Birch TW, Chick H, Martin CJ (1937) Experiments with pigs on a pellagra-producing diet. *Biochem J* 31 (11): 2065-2079.

Chick H, Macrae TF, Martin AJP, Martin CJ (1938a) Curative action of nicotinic acid on pigs suffering from the effects of a diet consisting largely of maize. *Biochem J* 32 (1): 10-12.

Chick H, Macrae TF, Martin AJ, Martin CJ (1938b) Experiments with pigs on a pellagra-inducing diet. II. *Biochem J* 32 (5): 844-854.

Chick H, Macrae TF, Martin AJP, Martin CJ (1938c) The water-soluble B-vitamins other than aneurin (vitamin B(1)), riboflavin and nicotinic acid required by the pig. *Biochem J* 32 (12): 2207-2224.

Chick H (1940) Nutritive value of white flour with vitamin B1 added and of wholemeal flour. *Lancet* 236 (6113): 511-512.

Chick H, El Sadr MM, Worden AN (1940) Occurrence of fits of an epileptiform nature in rats maintained for long periods on a diet deprived of vitamin B(6). *Biochem J* 34 (4): 595-600.

Chick H, Macrae TF, Worden AN (1940) Relation of skin lesions in the rat to deficiency in the diet of different B(2)-vitamins. *Biochem J* 34 (4): 580-594.

Chick H (1941) Nutritive value of bread. *Br Med J* 2 (4221) 790-791.

Chick H, Ellinger P (1941) The photosynthesizing action of buckwheat (*Fagopyrum esculentum*). *J Physiol* 100 (2): 212-230.

Chick H (1942) Biological value of the proteins contained in wheat flours. *Lancet* 239 (6188): 405-407.

Chick H, Cutting MEM (1943) Nutritive value of the nitrogenous substances in the potato: as measured by their capacity to support growth in young rats. *Lancet* 242 (6274): 667-669.

Martin C, Chick H, Hume M (1944) The British rations. Letter to the Editor of *The Times*, November 14, 1944

Chick H (1945) Nutritional researches in Vienna after the First World War. *Proc Nutr Soc* 3: 59-67.

Chick H, Slack EB (1945) Note on the nutritive value of the nitrogenous substances contained in dried yeast (*Torulopsis lipofera*). *Biochem J* 39 (2): 164-167.

Chick H, Copping (1945) Britain's National Bread in balanced nutrition. *The Scientific Monthly* 61 (3):226.

Chick H (1946) Nutritive value of proteins contained in wheat flours of different degrees of extraction. *Proc Nutr Soc* 4 (1): 6-9.

Chick H, Copping AM, Slack EB (1946) Nutritive values of wheat flours of different extraction rate. *Lancet* 247 (6389): 196-199.

Chick H, Slack EB (1946) Malted foods for babies: trials with young rats. *Lancet* 248 (6426): 601-603.

Chick H, Cutting ME (1947) Observation on the digestibility and nutritive value of the nitrogenous constituents of wheat bran. *Br J Nutr* 1 (2-3): 161-182.

Chick H (1947) Note on methods of determining the nutritive value of proteins. *Chemistry and Industry* 66 (June 7): 318-320.

Chick H, Slack EB (1948) Further observations on the nutritive value of the proteins contained in wheat flours of different extraction rates. *Br J Nutr* 2 (3): 205-213.

Chick H (1949) The Lister Institute of Preventive Medicine. *Endeavour* 8 (31): 106-111.

Chick H, Slack EB (1949) Distribution and nutritive value of the nitrogenous substances in the potato. *Biochem J* 45 (2): 211-221.

Chick H (1950) Supplementary nutritive values between the proteins of some common foods. *J Am Med Womens Assoc* 5 (11): 435-440.

Chick H (1951a) The aetiology of pellagra: a review of current theories. *J Trop Med Hygiene* 54 (10): 207-213.

Chick H (1951b) Nutritive value of vegetable proteins and its enhancement by admixture. *Br J Nutr* 5 (2): 261-265.

Chick H (1953) Early investigations of scurvy and the antiscorbutic vitamin. *Proc Roy Soc* 12 (3): 210-219.

Chick H (1954) The protein requirement of man. *Pharmazie* 9 (6): 452-455.

Chick H (1956) Charles James Martin, 1866-1955. *Biographical Memoirs of Fellows of the Royal Society* 2: 172-208.

Chick H, Hume M (1956) The work of the Accessory Food Factors Committee. *Br Med Bull* 12 (1): 5-8.

Chick H (1958) Wheat and bread: a historical introduction. *Proc Nutr Soc* 17 (1): 1-7.

Chick H, Peters AP (1969) Elmer Verner McCollum 1879-1967. *Biographical Memoirs of Fellows of the Royal Society* 15: 159-171.

Chick, Harriette; Hume, Margaret; and Macfarlane, Majorie (1971) *War on Disease. A History of the Lister Institute.* London: Andre Deutsch.

Chick H (1975) The discovery of vitamins. *Prog Food Nutr Sci* 1 (1): 1-20.

Chick H (1976) Study of rickets in Vienna 1919-1922. *Med Hist* 20 (1): 41-51.

Other Sources

Anon. (1942) *Brit Food J* 44(4) 31-40.

Anon. The wheatmeal loaf. *The Manchester Guardian*, March 23, 1942.

Anon. (1944) Meeting Report. *Proc Nutr Soc* 1 (1-2): 7-112

Anon. (1977) Harriette Chick obituary. *The Times of London*, July 11, 1977.

Barlow T (1883) On cases described as "acute rickets" which are probably a combination of scurvy and rickets, the scurvy being an essential, and the rickets a variable element. *Med-Chir Trans* 66: 159-220.

Baxby D (1908) The Chick-Martin test for disinfectants. *Epidemiol Infect* 133 (Suppl. 1) S13-S14.

Bland-Sutton J. (1889) *J Comp Med Surg* 10: 1

Blane, Gilbert (1785) *Observations of the Diseases Incident to Seamen*. London: Joseph Cooper.

Boas MA (1927) The effect of desiccation upon the nutritive properties of egg-white. *Biochem J* 21 (3): 712-724.

Boas Fixsen MA (1930) The biological values of proteins. II. The biological value of purified caseinogen and the influence of vitamin B2 upon biological values, determined by the balance sheet method. *Biochem J* 24 (6): 1794-1804.

Boas Fixsen MA, Jackson HM (1932) The biological values of proteins. III. A further note on the method used to measure the nitrogenous exchange of rats. *Biochem J* 26 (6): 1919-1922.

Boas Fixsen MA, Jackson HM (1932) The biological value of proteins. IV. The biological values of the proteins of wheat, maize and milk. *Biochem J* 26 (6): 1923-1933.

Boas-Fixsen MA, Hutchinson JCD, Jackson HM (1934) The biological values of proteins. V. The comparative biological values of the proteins of whole wheat, whole maize and maize gluten, measured by the growth of young rats. *Biochem J* 28 (2): 592-601.

Bollet AJ (1992) Politics and pellagra: the epidemic of pellagra in the U.S. in the early twentieth century. *Yale J Biol Med* 65 (3): 211-221.

Brock JF (1961) Dietary proteins in relation to man's health. *Fed Proc* 20 (1): 61-65.

Carpenter KJ (1983) The relationship of pellagra to corn and the low availability of niacin in cereals. In: J. Mauron, ed. *Nutritional Adequacy, Nutrient Availability and Needs* (Basel: Birlhauser Verlag), pp. 197-222.

Carpenter, Kenneth J (1986) *The History of Scurvy and Vitamin C.* Cambridge: Cambridge University Press.

Carpenter, Kenneth J (2000) *Beriberi, White Rice, and Vitamin B. A Disease, a Cause and a Cure.* Berkeley: University of California Press.

Carpenter KJ (2004) The Nobel Prize and the discovery of vitamins. <https://www.nobelprize.org/prizes/themes/the-nobel-prize-and-and-the-discovery-of-vitamins>

Carpenter KJ (2008) Harriette Chick and the problem of rickets. *J Nutrition* 138 (5): 827-832.

Casal, Don Gaspar (1762) *Historia natural, y medica de el Principado de Asturias.* Madrid: Martin. [Published in English translation in: Ralph H. Major, *Classic Descriptions of Disease, 3rd Ed.* (Springfield, IL: Charles C. Thomas, 1945), pp. 610-614.]

Chesney RW, Hedberg G (2010) Metabolic bone disease in lion cubs at the London Zoo in 1889: the original animal model of rickets. *Biomed Sci* 17 (Suppl 1): S36-S39.

Chick J (2014) Conversation with Jonathan Chick. *Addiction* 109: 1786-1793.

Chick J (2012) War on Disease: A History of the Lister Institute (book review). *Br Med J* 344: d8209.

Chittenden RH, Underhill FP (1917) The production in dogs of a pathological condition which closely resembles human pellagra. *Proc Natl Acad Sci USA* 3 (3): 195-197.

Cole T (2017) The remarkable life of Frances Wood. *Significance* https://

www.significancemagazine.com/science/563-the-remarkable-life-of-frances-wood

Cooper EA (1912) On the protective and curative properties of certain food-stuffs against polyneuritis induced in birds by a diet of polished rice. *J Hyg (Lond)* 12 (4): 436-462.

Cooper EA (1912) On the protective and curative properties of certain food-stuffs against polyneuritis induced in birds by a diet of polished rice. Part II. *J Hyg (Lond)* 14 (1):12-22.

Cooper S (1964) Snoek Piquante. In: Sissons, M., and French, P., eds., *The Age of Austerity* (Penguin Books: Middlesex, England), pp. 35-57.

Copping AM (1971) Sir Charles James Martin (1866-1955) *J Nutrition* 101 (1): 3-8.

Copping AM (1978) Obituary notice: Dame Harriette Chick. *Br J Nutr* 39 (1): 3-4.

Copping AM (1978) The history of the Nutrition Society. *Proc Nutr Soc* 37: 105-139.

Copping AM (1991) Dame Harriette Chick. In: *The Nutrition Society 1941-1991*, Elsie M. Widdowson, ed., (Oxford: CAB International), pp. 33-37.

Dean RFA (1951) The nutritional adequacy of a vegetable substitute for milk. *Br J Nutri* 5 (2): 269-274.

Drummond JC (1920) The nomenclature of the so-called accessory food factors (vitamins). *Biochem J* 14 (5): 660.

Dunn PM (1999) Professor Armand Trousseau (1801-67) and the treatment of rickets. *Arch Dis Child Fetal Neonatal Ed* 80: F155-F157.

Eijkman C (1929) Antineuritic vitamin and beriberi. Nobel lecture. In: *Nobel Lectures, Physiology or Medicine 1922-1941* Amsterdam: Elsevier, 1965. [Also available at https://www.nobelprize.org/prizes/medicine/1929/eijkman/lecture/]

Elvehjem CA, Koehn CJ, Oleson J (1936) A new essential dietary factor. *J Biol Chem* 115 (3): 707-719.

Elvehjem CA, Madden RJ, Strong FM, Woolley DW (1938) The isolation and identification of the anti-black tongue factor. *J Biol Chem* 123 (1): 137-149.

Fara, Patricia (2018) *A Lab of One's Own. Science and Suffrage in the First World War.* Oxford: Oxford University Press.

Funk C (1911) On the chemical nature of the substance which cures polyneuritis in birds induced by a diet of polished rice. *J Physiol* 43 (5): 395-400.

Funk C (1912) The etiology of the deficiency diseases. Beri-beri, polyneuritis in birds, epidemic dropsy, scurvy, experimental scurvy in animals, infantile scurvy, ship beri-beri, pellagra. *J State Med* 20: 341-368 [Reprinted in Goldblith, S. A., and Joslyn M. A., eds., *Milestones in Nutrition.* (Westport CT: Avi Publishing, 1964), pp. 145-172.]

Funk C (1913) Studies on pellagra. I. The influence of the milling of maize on the chemical composition and the nutritive value on maize-meal. *J. Physiol. (Lond.)* 47 (4-5): 389-392.

Goldberger J (1914) The etiology of pellagra. The significance of certain epidemiological observations with respect thereto. *Public Health Rep* 29 (26): 1683-1686.

Goldberger J, Waring CH (1915) The prevention of pellagra. A test of diet among institutional inmates. *Public Health Rep* 30 (43): 3117-3131.

Goldberger J, Wheeler GA (1915) Experimental pellagra in the human subject brought about by a restricted diet. *Public Health Rep* 30 (46): 3336-3339.

Goldberger J, Waring CH, Tanner WF (1923) Pellagra prevention by diet among institutional inmates. *Public Health Rep* 38 (41): 2361-2368.

Goldin, Claudia (2021) *Career & Family. Women's Century-Long Journey toward Equity.* Princeton: Princeton University Press.

Graham PA (1970) Women in academe. *Science* 169 (3952): 1284-1290.

Grijns G (1901) Over polyneuritis gallinarum. *Geneeskundig Tijdschrift voor Nererlandsch-Indië* 41: 3-110. [Published in English translation in: Grijns G (1935) *Researches on Vitamins 1900-1911* (Gorinchem: J Noorduyn en Zoon), pp. 1-108.]

Guy RA (1923) The history of cod liver oil as a remedy. *Am J Dis Child* 26 (2): 112-116.

Haines, Catherine M. C. (2001) *International Women in Science: A Biographical Dictionary to 1950* (Santa Barbara: ABC-CLIO), pp. 60-61.

Harte, Negley; North, John; and Brewis, Georgina (2019) *The World of UCL.* London: UCL Press'

Harvie, David I. (2002) *Limeys. The True Story of One Man's War against Ignorance, the Establishment and the Deadly Scurvy.* Stroud, U.K.: Sutton Publishing.

Heffer, Simon. (2021) *The Age of Decadence: Britain 1880 to 1914.* New York: Pegasus Books.

Henderson Smith A (1919) A historical inquiry into the efficacy of lime-juice for the prevention and cure of scurvy. *J Royal Med Corps* 32 (93-116): 188-208.

Hess AF, Unger LJ. (1917) Prophylactic therapy for rickets in a negro community. *J Amer Med Assn* 69 (19): 1583-1586.

Hess AF, Unger LJ (1921) The cure of infantile rickets by sunlight. *J Amer Med Assn* 77 (1): 39-41.

Holst A (1907) Experimental studies relating to "ship beri-beri" and scurvy: I. Introduction. *J Hyg (Lond)* 7 (5): 619-633.

Holst A, Frølich T (1907) Experimental studies relating to ship beri-beri and scurvy. II. On the etiology of scurvy. *J Hyg (Lond)* 7 (5): 634-671.

Hopkins FG (1912) Feeding experiments illustrating the importance of accessory factors in normal dietaries. *J Physiol* 44 (5-6): 425-460.

Huldschinsky K. (1919) Heilung von Rachitis durch Küntlich Höhensonne. *Deutsh Med Woch* 45: 712-713.

Hume EM (1944) Opportunities for nutritional research in the work of relief. *Proc Nutr Soc* 2 (3-4): 204-210.

Hume EM (1956) Obituary. Charles James Martin, Kt, C.M.G, F.R.C.P, D.Sc., F.R.S. (9 January 1866-15 February 1955) *Br J Nutr* 10 (1): 1-7.

Jackson, Lee (2014) *Dirty Old London: The Victorian Fight Against Filth*. New Haven: Yale University Press.

Kraut, Alan M. (2003) *Goldberger's War. The Life and Work of a Public Health Crusader*. New York: Hill and Wang.

Lind, James (1753) *A Treatise on the Scurvy*. Edinburgh: Kincaid and Donaldson.

Lind, James (1757) *An essay on the Most Effectual Means of preserving the Health of Seamen in the Royal Navy*. London: A. Millar.

Lunin N (1881) Über die Bedeutung der onorganischen Salze für Ernährung des Thieres. *Hoppe-Seyler Zeit f Physiol Chem* 5: 31-39.

Mackay HMM (1920) Observation on cases of rickets in an out-patient department. *Br Med J* 2 (3129): 929-932.

McCance RA, Widdowson EM (1942) Mineral metabolism of healthy adults on white and brown bread dietaries. *J Physiol* 101 (1): 44-85.

McCance, R. A., and Widdowson, E. M. (1956) *Breads White and Brown. Their Place in Thought and Social History*. London: Pitman.

McCollum, Elmer Verner (1957) *A History of Nutrition*. Boston: Houghton Mifflin.

McCollum EV, Davis M (1913) The necessity of certain lipins in the diet during growth. *J Biol Chem* 15 (1): 167-175.

McCollum EV, Davis M (1915) The nature of the dietary deficiencies of rice. *J Biol Chem* 23 (1): 181–230.

McCollum EV, Pitz W (1917) The "vitamin hypothesis" and deficiency diseases. *J Biol Chem* 31 (1): 229-253.

McCollum EV, Simmonds, N, Shipley PG, Park EA (1922) Studies on experimental rickets. Is there a substance other than fat-soluble A associated with certain fats which plays an important role in bone development? *J Biol Chem* 50 (1): 5-30.

McCollum EV, Simmonds N, Becker JE (1922) Studies on experimental rickets. XXI. An experimental demonstration of the existence of a vita-min which promotes calcium deposition. *J Biol Chem* 53 (2): 293-312.

Medical Research Committee. (1919) *Report on the present state of Knowledge concerning Accessory Food Factors (Vitamines)*. London, His Majesty's Stationery Office.

Medical Research Council. (1923) *Studies of Rickets in Vienna. 1919-22.* London: His Majesty's Stationary Office, 1923.

Medical Research Council. (1924) *Report on the Present State of Knowledge of Accessory Food Factors (Vitamins)*. London: His Majesty's Stationery Office.

Medical Research Council. (1932) *Vitamins: A Survey of Present Knowledge.* London: His Majesty's Stationery Office.

Medical Research Council (1940) Improved quality of bread. Higher extraction of flour. *Br Med J* 2 (4152): 164.

Medical Research Council (1941) National Flour for bread. MRC specifications. *Br Med J* 1 (4195): 828-829.

Medical Research Council (1951) *Studies of Undernutrition, Wuppertal 1946-9.* Medical Research Council Special Reports Series No. 275. London: His Majesty's Stationery Office.

Medical Research Council (1941) National flour. A second memorandum. *Lancet* 237 (6144): 703-704

Mellanby E (1918) The part played by an "accessory factor" in the production of experimental rickets. *Proc Physiol Soc* (January 26, 1918) xi-xii.

Mellanby, Edward (1921) *Experimental Rickets*. Medical Research Council Special Report No. 61. London: His Majesty's Stationery Office.

Mellanby EA (1918) Further demonstration of the part played by accessory food factors in the ætiology of rickets. *Proc Physiol Soc* (December 14, 1918) liii-liv.

Mellanby E (1920) Discussion of the importance of accessory food factors (vitamins) in the feeding of infants. *Proc Roy Soc Med* 13 (Sect Study Dis Child): 57-77.

Mellanby E (1930) The relation of diet to health and disease. *Br Med J* 1 (3614): 677-681.

Ministry of Food (1945) *Report of the Conference on the Post-War Loaf.* Cmd. 6701. London: H. M. Stationery Office.

Morrissey, S (1993) Dame Harriette Chick D.B.E. (1875-1977). In: Brindman, Lynn, ed., *Women Physiologists: An Anniversary Celebration of their Contributions to British Physiology* (London: Portland Press), pp. 21-29.

Owen I (1889) Geographical distribution of rickets, acute and subacute rheumatism, chorea, cancer, and urinary calculus in the British islands. *Br Med J* 1: 113-116.

O'Riodan JLH, Bijvoet OLM (2014) Rickets before the discovery of vitamin D. *BoneKEy Reports* 3: article number 478

Oxford Dictionary of National Biography. New York: Oxford University Press, 2004, pp. 409-410.

Reed P (2021) Alfred Fletcher's campaign for black smoke abatement, 1864–96: Anticipating the 1956 Clean Air Act. *Ine J Hist Engin Tech* DOI: 10.1080/17581206.2021.1985388. Available at: https://doi.org/10.1080/175 81206.2021.1985388.

Ross S (1962) *Scientist:* the story of a word. *Ann Science* 18 (2): 65-85.

Russell, Bertrand (1967) *The Autobiography of Bertrand Russell v. 1.* Boston: Little, Brown.

Sayer, Jane E (1973) *The Fountain Unsealed. A History of the Notting Hill and Ealing High School.* Welwyn Garden City: Broadwater Press.

Siler JF, Garrison PE, MacNeal WJ (1914) Pellagra: a summary of the first progress report of the Thompson-McFadden Pellagra Commission. *JAMA* 62 (1): 8 – 12.

Sitwell, William (1988) *Eggs or Anarchy.* New York: Simon and Schuster.

Tomlinson, Margaret (1985) *Three Generations in the Honiton Lace Trade.* Sidmouth: Sovereign Printing Group.

van Leersum EC (1926) The discovery of vitamins. *Science* 64 (1658): 357-358

Voss HE (1956) Nicolai Lunin—1853-1937. *J Amer Dietetic Assn* 32 (4): 317-320.

Walton JK (1979) Mad dogs and Englishmen: the conflict over rabies in late Victorian England. *J Social History* 13 (2): 219-239.

Widdowson EM (1992) Undernutrition in Germany in the post-war period. In: Widdowson, E. M., and Mathers, J., eds. *The Contributions of Nutrition to Human and Animal Health* (Cambridge: Cambridge University Press), pp. 293-302.

Widdowson EM (1936) A study of English diets by the individual method: Part I. Men. *J Hyg (Lond)* 36 (3): 269-292.

Widdowson EM, McCance RA (1936) A study of the English diets by the individual method. Part II. Women. *J Hyg Lond* 36 (3): 293-309.

Widdowson EM (1991) Dame Harriette Chick. In: *The Nutrition Society 1941-1991.* Widdowson, Elsie M., ed. (Oxford: C.A.B. International, 1991), p. 37.

Wiltshire HW (1918) A note on the value of germinated beans in the treatment of scurvy, and some points in prophylaxis. *Lancet* 192 (4972): 811-813.

Wilson EA (1905) The medical aspect of the *Discovery's* voyage to the Antarctic. *Br Med J* 2 (2323) 77-80.

Wilson LG (1975) The clinical definition of scurvy and the discovery of vitamin. *J Hist Med Allied Sci* 30 (1): 40-60.

Women in the Biochemical Society. Centre for the History of Medicine, University of Warwick. 10 November 2010. https://warwick.ac.uk/fac/arts/history/chm/research/womenbiochemists/biochemicalsociety

Wright, MD (1941) The nutritive value of bread. Fortified white flour and national wheatmeal compared. *Br Med J* 2 (4219) 689-692.

Zernike, Kate (1923) *The Exceptions. Nancy Hopkins, MIT, and the Fight for Women in Science.* New York: Scribner.

INDEX

www.ingramcontent.com/pod-product-compliance
Lightning Source LLC
Chambersburg PA
CBHW071243130626
46556CB00003B/1134